MAR 1 2 2012

Tell Me What to Eat If I Have Inflammatory Bowel Disease

Nutritional Guidelines for Crohn's Disease and Colitis

By Kimberly A. Tessmer, RD LD

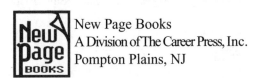

New Page Books
A Division of The Career Press, Inc.
Pompton Plains, NJ

Copyright © 2012 by Kimberly A. Tessmer, RD, LD

All rights reserved under the Pan-American and International Copyright Conventions. This book may not be reproduced, in whole or in part, in any form or by any means electronic or mechanical, including photocopying, recording, or by any information storage and retrieval system now known or hereafter invented, without written permission from the publisher, The Career Press.

TELL ME WHAT TO EAT IF I HAVE INFLAMMATORY BOWEL DISEASE
EDITED AND TYPESET BY KATHRYN HENCHES
Cover design by Lucia Rossman, Digi Dog Design
Printed in the U.S.A.

To order this title, please call toll-free 1-800-CAREER-1 (NJ and Canada: 201-848-0310) to order using VISA or MasterCard, or for further information on books from Career Press.

616.342

CAREER PRESS

New Page BOOKS

The Career Press, Inc.
220 West Parkway, Unit 12
Pompton Plains, NJ 07444
www.careerpress.com
www.newpagebooks.com

Library of Congress Cataloging-in-Publication Data

Tessmer, Kimberly A.
    Tell me what to eat if I have inflammatory bowel disease : nutritional guidelines for Crohn's disease and colitis /Kimberly Tessmer. -- 1
        p. cm.
    Includes bibliographical references and index.
    ISBN 978-1-60163-195-4 (pbk.) -- ISBN 978-1-60163-631-7 (ebook)
    1. Inflammatory bowel diseases--Popular works. 2. Inflammatory bowel diseases--Diet therapy--Recipes. 3. Self-care, Health--Popular works. I. Title.

RC862.I53T46 2012
616.3'44--dc23

2011037716

Dedication

I dedicate this book to all of those people out there that deal with IBD every day. I have learned so much by writing this book and have a much better idea of the challenges you face, and I praise you for the daily strength it takes. I hope this book is able to help you in some way. I also dedicate this book to my dad and my late mom whom I miss dearly. I thank them both for the gift they passed on to me of helping others. They have shown me all my life how important it is to be there and take care of each other. That is what gives me my passion to be a dietitian and help others deal with their struggles.

Acknowledgments

A loving thank you to my wonderful husband, Greg, who works so hard, which allows me to do what I love; and to my daughter, Tori, who was patient enough to give Mommy the time to do her writing. Thank you to *all* of my family and friends for your love, support, and encouragement. I would like to sincerely thank all of the health professionals who offered their advice, recommendations, and delicious recipes for this book. A special thank you to Kate Scarlata, RD, for use of her valuable information.

Disclaimer

At the time this book was written all information in this book was believed by the author to be correct and accurate. Information on inflammatory bowel disease changes frequently as more research is being completed. Always keep yourself up-to-date by reading reputable and current publications and speaking with your healthcare provider. The author shall have no liability of any kind for damages of any nature however caused. The author will not accept any responsibility for any omissions, misinterpretations, or mis-statements that may exist within this book. The author does not endorse any product or company listed in this book. Always consult with your healthcare provider for medical advice as well as recommendations on any type of supplement or herbal supplement you plan on taking. The author is not engaged in rendering medical services and this book should not be construed as medical advice, nor should it take the place of regular scheduled appointments with your healthcare provider and dietitian on a regular basis.

Contents

Introduction

Inflammatory Bowel Disease, or IBD, is a term that covers a complex group of diseases that tend to be difficult to diagnose and, at times, treat. Two of the most common forms of IBD are Crohn's disease and ulcerative colitis. That may sound like a lot of medical jargon, but in simpler terms IBD is a group of disorders that causes inflammation in the digestive tract. Though there are some similarities between Crohn's disease and ulcerative colitis there are also some major differences. One big difference is the area of the digestive tract that they affect. Ulcerative colitis mainly affects the large intestines (the colon) and the rectum, whereas Crohn's disease most commonly affects the small intestines and/or colon, though it can affect any part of the digestive tract.

IBD can affect people with varying degrees of intensity, symptoms, and illness. Although medications and, in some cases, surgery may be the treatment of choice, diet is another important element that should not be forgotten in the goal to help relieve symptoms, reduce the number of flare-ups, and restore quality of life. And the good news is that diet is one thing we *do* have control over.

With more than 1.4 million Americans thought to have IBD, people with this disease are hardly alone. As awareness of this disease grows so does the pool of resources, support groups, and current research. You don't have to go it alone, and there are steps you can take to help gain back some control of your life and your health.

This book serves just that purpose. This book will help people diagnosed with IBD better understand their disease and gain knowledge of what exactly they can do from a dietary and life-style standpoint. Not only will it provide insight to you, but also to family members and friends on whom you lean for support. You will find in this book practical information, diet advice, answers to your questions, useful information about supplements and other alternative treatments, helpful recipes, and more. My hope is that people with IBD will use this book to feel less helpless and more empowered about their life and health.

This book should not substitute, in any way, visits to your doctor and dietitian who specialize in these types of disorders. It should in no way be used as your only means of treating your disease. Instead, the book should be used as a complement to your medical teams instructions and advice and also used as a reference when needed.

Chapter 1

Everything You Ever Wanted to Ask Your Doctor About IBD

Are you one of almost 1.4 million Americans that suffer with inflammatory bowel disease- or what is better known as IBD? Do you question whether you or a loved one may have this disease? Have you been diagnosed but are still unsure as to what it is you really suffer from? To accept your disease and take part in managing your symptoms you first need to truly understand the nuts and bolts of this disease. This chapter will attempt to begin answering some of your most burning questions and clarify what you may have heard from your doctor but are having trouble getting a handle on. You will learn all of the most pertinent information on IBD in this chapter and throughout this book.

? How does the digestive tract function?

Because both forms of IBD lie somewhere within the digestive tract it is essential to understand the basics of the digestive system to understand IBD. Our digestive system includes the mouth, esophagus, stomach, small intestines, large intestines (also referred to as the colon), and rectum. Other organs such as the liver, pancreas, and gallbladder are not considered part of the digestive tract buy play essential roles in the digestive process. This delicate yet resilient system of organs has the crucial job of breaking down and converting food into nutrients that the body can then absorb into the bloodstream to fuel the body's cells, allowing us to survive. Our digestive system usually doesn't get the kudos it deserves for all the essential work it does. In fact, we hardly pay attention to our digestive system unless something goes awry, as in the case with IBD.

The digestive process begins way at the top in your mouth and ends in the small intestines. When we smell those wonderful aromas of our favorite foods we start to salivate in preparation for that first bite of food. The mouth, stomach, and small intestines contain an inside lining called the mucosa. The mucosa contains tiny glands that produce juices necessary for the digestion and breaking down of food. The digestive tract is also made up of a layer of smooth muscle that aids in the breaking down and movement of food along the digestive tract.

Tip

Why is the whole digestion process so vitally important to our body? No matter how healthy a food is, it is not in a form our body can use for nourishment. Through digestion foods must be changed into smaller molecules of nutrients before they can be absorbed into the bloodstream and carried to waiting cells for nourishment and energy.

After food enters the mouth it heads down the throat and esophagus and into the awaiting stomach. The stomach has three major tasks in the digestion process. First, it houses the food that has been swallowed. Second, it mixes up the food, liquid, and digestive juices (including acids and enzymes) that the stomach produces, and last, the stomach empties its contents slowly into the small intestines.

The small intestines is made up of three parts: the duodenum, the jejunum, and the ileum, which is the final section leading into the large intestines. The inner walls of the small intestines are enveloped with villi, small finger-like projections through which nutrients are absorbed into the body. Every piece of food we put in our mouth is broken down into absorbable nutrients including carbohydrates, protein, fats, vitamins, and minerals. Through specific enzymes, protein is broken down into amino acids, starches to simple sugars, and fats into fatty acids and glycerol. Even the water in foods finds its way into the bloodstream to help meet the body's fluids needs.

Tip Carbohydrates spend the least amount of time within the stomach while protein lasts a bit longer and fats stay the longest.

The food continues on its digestive journey, dissolving into the enzymes and juices produced by the liver, pancreas, and intestines, being pushed ahead to allow further digestion. From there, the digested nutrients are finally absorbed through the walls of the small intestines and transported throughout the body to where they are needed. The next stop is the large intestines. By this time the absorption of nutrients is just about finished. The function of the large intestines is to remove water from undigested matter and to form solid waste that can be expelled from the body.

Tip The organs of the digestive tract are also known as the alimentary canal. An adult's digestive tract runs about 30 feet long.

? What is IBD?

Inflammatory bowel disease (IBD) is an umbrella term used for several chronic conditions that cause inflammation in various parts of the digestive tract, specifically the intestines. The exact symptoms and type of condition depends on which part of the digestive tract is involved. The two major forms of IBD include Crohn's disease and ulcerative colitis. Both of these forms of IBD have one common feature and that is the abnormal response by the body's immune system. Normally our immune system protects our body from things such as infection. In people with IBD, the immune system doesn't react as it should. Instead it essentially attacks certain parts of the intestines. The attack of the immune system sends white blood cells into the lining of the intestines, where chronic inflammation is the result. These cells ultimately generate harmful by-products that lead to ulceration and injury to the bowel and that, in turn, causes the symptoms of IBD.

? What is the difference between Crohn's disease and ulcerative colitis?

The biggest different between these two forms of IBD, Crohn's disease and ulcerative colitis, is which part of the intestines is affected. Crohn's disease can occur in any part of the digestive system but most commonly affects the lower part of the small intestines, called the ileum, and sometimes the first part of the large intestines. Ulcerative colitis affects only the large intestines, specifically the lining of the rectum and colon.

? How does IBD affect the digestive process?

We know the basic workings of the digestive process and we know that IBD occurs somewhere along the digestive tract. The problem lies in the fact that when the small intestines becomes inflamed, as in Crohn's disease, it cannot efficiently absorb the nutrients needed for the body from the food you eat. Many of these nutrients are instead excreted from the body without ever being absorbed. In addition, the undigested food that moves into the large intestines makes water absorption more difficult, which can cause diarrhea. This can leave people with Crohn's disease very nutrient deficient, causing all type of problems we will discuss later in the book. Because ulcerative colitis doesn't affect the small intestines, nutrients are correctly absorbed like they should be, however, inflammation in the large intestines keeps it from absorbing water, causing diarrhea and other symptoms.

? How is IBD diagnosed?

A thorough health history and physical exam are first on the list. Then if your doctor suspects you have IBD you will need to have a combination of tests performed to confirm your doctor's suspicions. You will need to be patient as it can take a while for your doctor to diagnose IBD, because the symptoms vary and can be quite similar to many other digestive conditions. Diagnosing IBD involves determining the disease type, the extent of the disease, and any complications that may be associated with it.

Tests performed might include many of the following:

- **Blood tests:** to test for signs of anemia, inflammation, infection, specific antibodies, electrolyte levels, and liver function.

- **Stool sample:** to test for bacterial infection that can trigger flare-ups as well as for signs of bleeding.

- **Colonoscopy:** allows the doctor to see the entire lining of the large intestines and the very last part of the small intestines to pinpoint inflammation, bleeding, and/or ulcers. A biopsy may also be taken.

- **Sigmoidoscopy:** allows the doctor to see the lining of the lower part of the large intestines to pinpoint inflammation, bleeding, and/or ulcers. A biopsy may also be taken.

- **EGD (Esophagogastroduodenoscopy):** allows the doctor to examine the lining of the esophagus, stomach, and first part of the small intestines to look for damage. A biopsy may also be taken.

- **Endoscopy with capsule:** allows the doctor to examine the entire small intestines through a small pill-shaped camera that is swallowed.

- **X-rays with barium:** barium coats the lining of the digestive tract while x-rays are taken, allowing the doctor to check for signs of IBD.

- **CAT scan:** takes x-rays of the body, allowing the doctor to look for signs of ulcerative colitis.

Magnetic Resonance Imaging (MRI) and ultrasound are other testing measures used quite frequently.

This may seem like a long list of tests and you may not go through all of them, but keep in mind that it is essential that your doctor confirms an accurate diagnosis of your particular disease in order to prescribe a treatment that will be effective for you and help to relieve your symptoms. Even after you have been properly diagnosed and your disease type is determined, you will still need to periodically undergo some of these tests. These tests are valuable tools in determining whether your treatment plan is working and to catch any complications that may arise early.

? What are the symptoms of IBD?

Although Crohn's disease and ulcerative colitis share a few of the same symptoms, many are quite different. In addition, symptoms tend to vary among individuals, and their severity depends on the severity of an individual's condition.

The symptoms experienced with Crohn's disease depend highly on the location and the severity of the inflammation within the gastrointestinal tract.

For Crohn's disease symptoms may include:

- Abdominal pain.
- Diarrhea.
- Weight loss/loss of appetite.
- Fatigue.
- Growth failure or failure to thrive in children.
- Fever.
- Anemia.
- Rectal bleeding.

Being that ulcerative colitis mainly affects the large intestines, most symptoms are due to inflammation, damage, and ulceration of the delicate lining in that area.

For ulcerative colitis symptoms may include:

- Frequent and bloody diarrhea.
- Abdominal pain and cramping.
- increased intestinal gas.

- Fatigue.
- Weight loss/loss of appetite.
- Rectal urgency.
- Rectal bleeding.
- Anemia.
- Joint pain.
- Growth failure or failure to thrive in children.

? What is the treatment for IBD?

Once your doctor has confirmed IBD and determined the type you have, a treatment plan will be developed. Keeping in mind that each individual's case will differ, your treatment plan will take into account your symptoms and how severe they are, which part of your digestive tract is being affected and whether you have other health problems not dealing with the digestive system. What works for one person with IBD may not be what works for another. Your treatment might go through a trial and error period, especially with medications, until your doctor finds what works best for you.

Depending on your individual case, treatment for IBD may include a combination of the following:

- Medications (to reduce inflammation, relieve symptoms, and prevent flare-ups).
- Surgery (usually for severe IBD when medications do not help).
- Dietary modifications.
- Nutritional supplements.
- Lifestyle changes including stress reduction and getting plenty of sleep.

It may benefit you to keep a journal of medications, dietary changes, and other treatments that are implemented to help you keep track of any side effects as well as positive and negative effects. This will help keep your doctor more informed about what is and what is not helping.

Tip	Do not take over-the-counter medication to relieve symptoms such as diarrhea or pain without first speaking with your doctor. For people with IBD these medications may make symptoms worse.

Experts are continuing to study many new treatments for managing symptoms of IBD, such as new medications, biologic therapies, fish and flaxseed oils, and probiotics. Clinical studies are ongoing, and you can find out more if you are interested in participating by visiting the clinical trials Website of the U.S. National Institutes of Health at *www.clinicaltrials.gov*.

? Will my IBD ever go away?

Unfortunately the answer to this question, at this point in time, is no. IBD is a chronic condition and people with this disease need to seek treatment throughout their lives. However, most people with IBD may experience remission, meaning they can go for a prolonged period of time with few to no symptoms. People with IBD are considered in remission when their bowel is functioning normally and the symptoms of IBD are no longer bothersome. Remission is the goal of treatment for all people with IBD. Most people with IBD will experience bouts of flare-ups, when the disease and its symptoms are active, and periods of remission throughout their lives.

? What causes IBD?

The cause of IBD is presently unknown. Some experts believe that the abnormal reaction of an individual's immune system to treat bacteria, food, and other substances as foreign in the digestive tract may trigger IBD. The theory is that the immune system's response is to attack these foreign bodies, which in turn causes white blood cells to accumulate in the intestinal lining, producing chronic inflammation. However, scientists are still testing this theory to try to figure out if this abnormal response of the immune system is a cause of the disease or a result of it. Some believe it is a virus or bacterium that may trigger IBD; others have looked at the possibility that the inflammation may be a result of an autoimmune response or environmental issues.

Experts have also considered that certain genes may cause the immune system to overreact and contribute to the cause of IBD, especially ulcerative colitis. There may not be a definitive answer as to what causes IBD, though research is continuing, but experts have definitely agreed as to what does *not* cause IBD. Years ago they thought that stress and eating certain foods were main culprits, but they now know this is not the case. However, both of these factors have been known to worsen symptoms in people with IBD.

? How serious is IBD and are there other potential complications?

IBD is a very serious chronic condition, and living with it can be difficult at times. Not just flare-ups but serious medical complications can occur as a result of having IBD. Some people experience mild disease symptoms or flare-ups, whereas others can be almost incapacitated by the severity of their symptoms.

Proper treatment, both medical and dietary, as well as learning to emotionally cope with your condition, should be on the top of your priority lists and is the key to helping manage your disease.

IBD can be the source of other complications outside of the intestinal tract, or what is referred to as *extraintestinal,* including anemia (due to loss of blood within the digestive tract), arthritis and joint pain, osteoporosis, inflammation in the eye and other eye problems, liver and kidney problems, skin conditions, and growth problems in children. Some of these problems seem to be caused from poor absorption of nutrients and others may be due to inflammation. If these conditions are a problem, there is a chance that some of them may get better as IBD is treated. However, some of them must be treated separately.

Some potential intestinal complications of IBD can happen in both Crohn's disease and ulcerative colitis. However, the majority of them are disease specific, meaning they occur exclusively in one form of IBD or the other.

- Toxic megacolon can be life threatening but is something that is relatively rare. It typically occurs more in elderly patients than in younger ones and in colitis patients more then in Crohn's patients, and involves massive distention of the colon.

- Small intestinal bacterial overgrowth (SIBO) is a condition that can occur in both Crohn's and ulcerative colitis. It occurs when excessive amounts of bacteria are found in the small intestines and usually resolves after a course of antibiotic treatment.

- Rupture of the bowel can occur in both forms of IBD. It can occur when chronic inflammation and ulceration weakens the intestinal walls to the point that a hole or rupture develops. This can cause serious infection.

Potential intestinal complications of Crohn's disease:

- Abscesses are caused by deep ulcers and can cause localized infection caused by bacteria.

- Strictures are scars that cause narrowing of the intestinal walls. These strictures are not a problem unless they cause a bowel obstruction.

- Fistulas are caused by ulcers within the intestinal tract that can turn into channels or tracts called fistulas joining one part of the intestines to another part or to another organ. These abnormal paths often become infected.

- Malnutrition may not be an intestinal disorder but it begins in the intestines. Because Crohn's disease affects the small intestines, which is the part of the digestive system that absorbs the most nutrients, malnutrition or a deficiency of nutrients can occur.

Potential intestinal complications of ulcerative colitis:

- Fulminant colitis affects a small number of people with colitis and involves damage to the entire thickness of the intestinal wall resulting in a condition called ileus. It is even more rare in Crohn's disease.

Some of these complications, for both forms of IBD are rare, but others can be quite common so if you notice a change in your symptoms alert your doctor immediately.

? If I have IBD am I at a higher risk for colon cancer?

People with IBD are only at a slightly higher risk of ending up with cancer of the colon or large intestines. At this point in time the link seems to be stronger with ulcerative colitis than with Crohn's disease, but research suggests that Crohn's patients are at an increased risk as well. For IBD in general the risk of colon cancer seems to depend on how long the individual has had IBD and how much of the colon is affected by the disease. In addition, people who have family members with colon cancer increase their risk even more. People with IBD should discuss with their doctor when they should begin being checked for colon cancer, what tests need to be done, and how often. The earlier cancer is found the easier it is to cure and treat.

? Does IBD have a genetic link?

This can be a more difficult question than it may seem. Both forms of IBD, Crohn's disease and ulcerative colitis, do appear to run in families, though Crohn's disease seems to have a higher tendency. It is estimated that about 10 to 20 percent of people with Crohn's disease have at least one family member (brothers, sisters, children, and parents) with the disease. But that means a good 80 to 90 percent of people do not have a family history of IBD. If they do have a family member with IBD it isn't always an immediate family member such as a parent or sibling and can sometimes be an extended family member. The genetic link doesn't appear to be as simple as the passing of the disease from parent to child.

It has also been discovered that Crohn's disease tends to be diagnosed at an earlier age in people who have relatives with IBD. Studies continue to try to better isolate the exact genes that carry the trigger for IBD. Clearly at this point in time the genetic link is not yet well understood.

? Who gets IBD?

It appears that both males and females are equal partners when it comes to IBD, as it seems to occur in both genders at roughly the same rate. IBD is first seen mostly in the age group between 20 and 40 years old, though first symptoms can show up as early as the teen years. However, it can be found in children over the age of 5 as well and is not unheard of for older individuals in their 50s and 60s to experience the onset of IBD. Although IBD has been observed throughout all ethnic groups, it seems to have the highest incidence within the Jewish population of European descent. In addition, Caucasians seem to also have an increased risk of developing IBD.

? Will having IBD affect my chances of becoming pregnant or carrying a healthy baby?

If you suffer with ulcerative colitis your chances of becoming pregnant are the same as for women without the disease. The same holds true for Crohn's disease if you are in remission. However, if you are having flare-ups with Crohn's disease you may have a little more trouble. Many health professionals agree that you should be in remission for at least six months before trying to conceive.

If you are thinking of trying to conceive you should speak with your doctor first. Some medications may not be safe if you do become pregnant. However, never stop taking medications if you do become pregnant without your doctor's knowledge. Stopping medications may cause flare-ups and make it more difficult to get your disease back under control.

? What type of doctor diagnoses and treats IBD and other digestive disorders?

If you are experiencing what you believe are recurring digestive symptoms, as the ones previously outlined, your best bet is to seek out an expert in this field. Doctors specializing in this area are *gastroenterologists*. These doctors specialize in treating and diagnosing conditions of the entire gastrointestinal or digestive tract.

The first step in understanding and treating IBD is to work with a gastroenterologist that will help to diagnose your symptoms. Feeling comfortable and confident with the doctor you choose is vitally important to your well-being. You may consider asking your primary doctor for a referral and/or asking friends and family for possible suggestions. The quicker you find a specialist you are comfortable with, the quicker you can get to the bottom of your symptoms and begin treatment.

To get the most from your visit with your doctor, try following a few of these tips:

- Find out ahead of time how much time your doctor will be able to allocate to your visit, especially if this is your first meeting with the doctor. You want to be sure you have plenty of time to have all of your questions and concerns addressed. If you think you will need more time than is allotted, then speak up and ask for that time.

- Describe the symptoms you are feeling in as much detail as possible. They may not be the easiest symptoms to discuss, but the more detailed you are, the better understanding your doctor will have about your condition. Keep in mind that this is the doctor's specialty and he or she has heard symptoms like this many times before.

- Bring an updated, written list of your medications and their doses to your appointment.

- Take the time to write down a list of questions you have before your appointment. Prioritize your list from most important to least important to ensure you take care of the questions that are causing you the most concern. Many times the doctor's answer to your most pressing questions will also answer other questions further down on your list. And remember that *no* question is trivial. If you have a concern then it *is* important! If you are diagnosed with IBD it will be your job to stay as well informed about your disease and treatments options as possible and advocate for your own health.

- Don't be afraid to jot down notes as the doctor is answering your questions or discussing other issues with you. Your doctor may be giving you treatment options that you will want to think about before making a decision, and you will want to refer to your notes first.

- If at all possible bring a family member or friend to your appointment with you. He or she can help to provide emotional support and act as a back-up to all of the information you will be receiving.

? What types of questions should I ask my doctor?

These are just a few examples of questions you may want to ask your doctor. As you read through these and the remainder of the book, you should get a much better idea of the questions you will need to ask. It might be helpful to make notes to yourself as you read through.

Could there be another condition other then IBD causing my symptoms? Because the symptoms of IBD can mimic those of so many other digestive conditions, it is important to ask your doctor this question. In addition, there are other conditions that can be caused by IBD so you want to be sure all of your symptoms are addressed.

What form of IBD do I have? Once you are diagnosed with IBD you should ask your doctor which form you have, Crohn's disease or ulcerative colitis, and make certain you understand the difference. They are both collectively known as IBD but require different forms of treatments, because they affect different parts of the digestive tract.

What treatment and/or medication will you recommend and why? Treatment for either form of IBD is very individualized, so you will want to find out what is right for you. In addition, because IBD can cause other conditions such as weight loss or anemia, you may need treatment for these as well. You will also want to know if the medications you will be taking can cause any side effects.

When will I start to feel better? One of your main goals will be to get your symptoms under control, so you will want to ask your doctor how long it will take for your specific treatment to take effect and when you should start to see improvements. It is important to be aware of this time frame and to ask what the next step will be if you don't start to feel better when expected. Waiting too long to try something different can cause more damage and cause you more misery.

Are there changes to my diet I should make? This is a great question and one that we will address in many of the chapters throughout this book. Dietary changes can be very beneficial as an additional treatment for IBD. You should ask your doctor for a referral to a registered dietitian that specializes in digestive disorders to learn which dietary changes will be beneficial to your individual condition.

Which symptoms should I be concerned about the most? Because IBD is a chronic disorder there will be symptoms you deal with on a recurring basis. Not all of these symptoms will require a special trip to the doctor's office but some may. Ask your doctor at what point he or she would like you to come in if your symptoms changes or you experience new ones.

Are there other lifestyle changes that will help ease my symptoms? For people with chronic diseases, such as IBD, other lifestyle changes such as getting enough sleep, exercise, healthy eating, stress management, and smoking cessation may help to increase energy and prevent flare-ups. However, in some cases, certain foods and activities may need to be limited. Ask your doctor what lifestyle changes would benefit you most and if there are any limitations to your individual case.

What type of regular monitoring will I need? IBD requires regular monitoring to assess whether your treatment is effective and to watch for any complications and/or related conditions that can arise. Ask your doctor what tests you will need on a regular basis and how often so that you are prepared. In addition you will want to know what these complications and/or related conditions might include.

Chapter 2

Discovering Other Digestive Disorders

Digestive problems are one of the most common conditions that affect Americans today. Many types of digestive problems can exist, with several of the symptoms mimicking each other closely. The symptoms of IBD can be quite similar to those of IBS (irritable bowel syndrome), diverticulosis, and celiac disease, just to name a few. Because symptoms can be so similar, this chapter will look a little more closely at these other digestive disorders.

IBS Is Not the Same as IBD

One of the digestive disorders most confused with IBD is IBS. The abbreviations look quite similar, and the symptoms can be as well, but IBS is much different from IBD. IBS is much more prevalent than IBD, with an estimated 50 million people, mostly women, being affected. IBS does not cause inflammation or damage to the intestines or other parts of the digestive system, and in addition does not lead to other health problems, as is the case with IBD. IBS is a syndrome and is not a disease as IBD is (with syndrome meaning involving a group of symptoms).

IBS Info

IBS is a disorder that interferes with the normal functioning of the colon. Like IBD, experts are not quite sure what causes IBS. However, they do know that the nerves and muscles in the bowel appear to be extra sensitive in individuals with IBS, which most likely brings on the symptoms. People with IBS are more sensitive to things that might not bother other people, such as certain foods, large meals, stress, caffeine, medications, or alcohol. IBS is diagnosed when symptoms are absent of any other medical explanation.

The most common symptoms of IBS include abdominal pain or discomfort that is often reported as cramping, bloating, gas, diarrhea (which can be chronic), and/or constipation. These symptoms may not sound out of the ordinary and can many times be experienced by all types of people, depending on foods eaten, overeating, and so on. But if these symptoms are chronic or interfere with normal activities, there is most likely a problem and you should be looked at immediately. IBS has no cure but there are treatments that can help to relieve symptoms. Treatment can involve dietary changes, medications, and stress relief. The most effective treatment comes from working with your doctor to find the plan that works best for you.

IBS and diet

For many people with IBS, changes in diet can help to reduce symptoms, though that is easier said than done. When it comes to diet, every individual with IBS is unique in that they deal with different foods that may trigger symptoms. In addition, dietary modifications also depend on what your major symptoms are, and that, too, differs from person to person. Some people deal with chronic diarrhea while others may deal with constipation as their major culprit.

The best method of defense is to keep a food diary that includes foods you eat, as well as your symptoms and feelings for a few weeks to find out which foods trigger or aggravate your symptoms or make them worse. From there, you can take your notes to a registered dietitian, who can help you create an individualized meal plan that will help you to better manage your symptoms. It is important to see an expert and to not begin removing whole food groups from your diet. Just because one or two fruits or vegetables aggravate your symptoms, it doesn't mean all of them will. If, for instance, dairy foods seem to cause you problems, it may be because you just need to eat less of them, consume them with meals, or choose one, such as yogurt, that is better tolerated. If you need to avoid foods such as dairy products you will need to replace the nutrients specific to that food group by substituting other foods and/or taking supplements. Again, a dietitian can help you manage these important dietary changes the proper way.

Although each person with IBS is unique regarding which foods he or she can or cannot tolerate, in general, foods and ingredients that can worsen symptoms for a majority of people include:

- High fat/fried foods.
- Spicy foods.
- Milk products.
- Chocolate.
- Alcohol.
- Caffeinated beverages.
- Carbonated beverages.
- Gas-producing beans and vegetables.
- Sorbitol (an artificial sweetener used in sugar-free candy and gums).

For some people, especially those with constipation problems, adding more fiber, especially soluble fibers, such as beans, oats, psyllium, and certain fruits and vegetables, can help to alleviate some symptoms. Yet for others with more sensitive digestive nerves, more fiber can create more abdominal discomfort. Adding too much fiber too quickly can also easily cause gas and trigger symptoms in someone with IBS. We will discuss more about fiber later in the book.

It isn't always food alone that triggers symptoms but how much food is consumed in one meal, how many trigger foods you eat in one day, how quickly you eat, or even how much stress you are under while you eat. Eating four to five small, well-planned meals, instead of less frequent larger meals, can certainly help, along with paying attention to the types of foods you eat. In addition, drink plenty of water daily. This is especially important if you are increasing fiber intake or have chronic diarrhea, which can cause dehydration.

The FODMAP Dietary Approach

Another dietary approach that most people have probably not heard of but is used by nutrition experts to help treat IBS is called FODMAP. What are FODMAPs? FODMAP is an acronym for Fermentable, Oligo-, Di, and Mono-saccharides, and Polyols. FODMAPS are a group of fermentable short-chain carbohydrates that are believes to cause symptoms such as gas, bloating, and watery diarrhea for some IBS suffers. These FODMAP carbohydrates include lactose, fructose, fructans, sugar alcohols, and galactans (or GOS). Experts have found that normal functioning of the gastrointestinal (GI) tract is greatly influenced by two things: the bacterial flora that live within the gut and the food we consume. It has been found that these two factors are linked, because the food we consume affects the bacterial flora that reside within our GI tracts. The way FODMAPs come into play is that they are the carbohydrates that are the most prone to fermentation by this bacterial flora in our guts, which cause symptoms such as cramping, diarrhea, bloating, and gas—prime symptoms of IBS.

For this dietary approach you work with a physician and/or dietitian to eliminate all foods that contain these types of carbohydrates for a trial period of around one or two weeks. If FODMAP carbs were causing your symptoms it would be evident by relief of symptoms in just a few days; FODMAP carbs are slowly and individually added back to the diet one at a time to find out which ones are causing problems and which ones are well tolerated. The goal is to only eliminate types of carbs that cause symptoms for that individual so he or she can follow a liberal and varied diet. Even if a FODMAP is found to cause problems, many people can still tolerate it in smaller doses. The FODMAP approach can be complicated, but if an individual is willing to try, it can be quite useful in keeping symptoms under control. We will talk about this approach in Chapter 3, because it has also been shown to be functional in particular cases of IBD.

For more detailed information about IBS, check out *Tell Me What to Eat if I Have Irritable Bowel Syndrome*, by Elaine Magee, MPH, RD.

Diving Into Diverticular Disease

Yet another digestive disorder that can mimic the symptoms of IBD is diverticular disease, which mainly affects the colon. Diverticular disease includes *diverticulosis* and *diverticulitis*. Diverticulosis is the condition of having diverticula. Diverticula are small pouches of sacs that form in the wall of the colon (large intestines) that have abnormally bulged outward through weak spots. This condition occurs more often after the age of 40 and is found in more than half of Americans older than age 60. Diverticulitis occurs when these pouches or diverticula become inflamed or infected within the intestinal wall. Sometimes a small tear can also appear in the diverticula, and, if it is too large, infection and inflammation inside the abdomen can occur.

Diverticular disease info

If diverticulosis is discovered, it is mainly treated with a high-fiber diet and pain relievers if symptoms occur. Depending on the severity, a mild case of diverticulitis is treated with antibiotics to knock out the infection along with a liquid diet and/or low-fiber foods for a planned amount of time to help rest and heal the colon. In severe diverticulitis attacks, an individual may need to be hospitalized.

> **Tip**
>
> A popular diet myth surrounding diverticular disease is that eating nuts, seeds, corn, and popcorn will increase a person's risk of developing diverticulitis by getting caught in the diverticula. It is not necessary to eliminate these foods, but do remember to chew your food well.

Some experts believe that in addition to older age being a common factor and cause of diverticulitis, a low-fiber diet may also play a role. A high-fiber diet along with plenty of fluid and regular exercise may help to prevent the development of diverticulosis, may reduce symptoms in individuals who have diverticulosis, and may help prevent complications such as diverticulitis. Speak with a dietitian about learning how to get plenty of fiber in your diet. If you can't seem to get all you need through food, you can speak with your doctor about utilizing fiber supplements. Keep in mind that when adding fiber to your diet, it is important to do it slowly and to drink plenty of water along the way.

As with other digestive disorders, people differ in the amounts and type of foods they can safely consume before symptoms may occur. Keeping a food journal can help to identify foods that may cause or aggravate your symptoms. Your diet plan should be based on what works best for you. Because some of the symptoms of this condition can mimic those of other digestive disorders, see your doctor if you experience them and they persist so that you can be properly diagnosed and treated.

Research continues on the condition of diverticular disease in many areas, but most interesting is the research being done on a possible link between diverticular disease and IBD.

Uncovering Celiac Disease

The list continues with yet another digestive disorder that includes symptoms that, again, can mimic those of IBD. Celiac disease may be one that you have heard of because of its ties to a popular diet trend called a gluten-free diet, not to mention that celiac disease is more prevalent now than ever before. In fact, it is believed that more than 2 million Americans, or about one out of every 133 people, have the disease. Why is it more prevalent now? Most likely because the disease is gaining recognition, and methods of diagnosing the disease are improving as technology advances. This is good news for anyone experiencing the harsh symptoms that untreated and/or undiagnosed celiac disease can cause.

Tip

If you believe you have the symptoms mentioned in the following section, it is vitally important to see your doctor to be properly diagnosed. Never start a diet through self-diagnosis. So many digestive problems have symptoms that mimic each other and each condition has its own treatment plan. Starting on the wrong treatment plan can cause further delay of a diagnosis as well as cause further complications.

Celiac disease info

Celiac disease is an autoimmune inflammatory disorder of the small intestines that, at present time, has no cure. It is a disease that can affect both men and women as well as children, and most likely has some type of genetic link. People with celiac disease have a very different treatment (plan than those with IBD, IBS, or diverticular disease do. These people need a very special diet for life, which is the only form of treatment at this time. That diet is a 100-percent gluten-free diet. For people with celiac disease, consuming a food or beverage that contains any amount of gluten causes their bodies to produce specific antibodies that attack the small intestines. These antibodies destroy the villi within the lining of the small intestines as well as digestive enzymes. Once the villi in the small intestines is destroyed, the body loses its ability to absorb nutrients needed for good health such as carbohydrates, protein, fat, vitamins, minerals, and other essential, disease-fighting phytonutrients. Nutritional deficiencies along with the destruction of the lining of the small intestines can lead to numerous GI symptoms as well as serious health conditions, both short and long term.

Because the symptoms of celiac disease mimic those of so many other digestive conditions such as IBS and IBD, it fairly common for it to be misdiagnosed or for diagnosis to take some time. A simple blood test will tell your doctor if suspicion of celiac disease is present and further testing needs to be completed. Symptoms can include any of the following:

- Reoccurring abdominal bloating and pain.
- Pale and foul-smelling stool.
- Nausea and vomiting.
- Diarrhea.
- Constipation.
- Chronis alternating diarrhea with constipation.
- Excessive flatulence.

- Bone or joint pain.
- Muscle cramps.
- Weight loss.
- Depression.
- Iron deficiency with or without unexplained anemia.
- Failure to thrive in children.

Other health conditions that can occur secondary to celiac disease include lactose intolerance, osteoporosis, tooth enamel defects, central and peripheral nervous system disease, pancreatic disease, vitamin K deficiency associated with an increased risk for hemorrhaging, organ disorders such an amenorrhea, miscarriage, and infertility. People who have celiac disease and who do not adhere strictly to a gluten-free diet stand a greater chance of developing cancer in the intestinal and gastrointestinal areas as well.

Once a person with celiac disease begins a gluten-free diet, the tissues of the small intestines begin to heal, and associated symptoms begin to diminish. However, just because the intestine heals, it doesn't mean the person can stop following a gluten-free diet. Any ingestion of gluten will start the destruction all over again so a gluten-free diet needs to be followed closely for a lifetime.

Celiac disease and the gluten-free diet

Gluten is a protein found in wheat, rye, barley, and any derivative of these grains, so gluten-free foods are considered foods that are void of these proteins. Foods that are naturally gluten-free as well as healthy include fresh fruits and vegetables, potatoes, rice, legumes, poultry, meats, and fish. The key is being careful to prepare these foods without other gluten-containing products. Most dairy products are also gluten-free and only cause a problem if you are lactose intolerant. In addition to naturally gluten-free fresh foods, there are now a large variety of specially made gluten-free foods on the market such as cereals, muffins, breads, pastas, snacks, soups, and many more. Many restaurants have also joined the gluten-free train and have special menu items that are deemed gluten-free. That may not sound too bad, but believe me when I say that it takes a good dose of education from a health professional such as a registered dietitian to follow a gluten-free diet properly due to its complexity. A dietitian can also ensure that your gluten-free diet is healthy and well balanced. Gluten sneaks into foods in ways you would never think, and most of this time the word *gluten* is not a part of the offending ingredient. Learning how to label read and recognize gluten-containing ingredients along with further education is the diet for life to help avoid serious symptoms and health problems down the line, so for these people it is not a choice, but a way of life.

Celiac disease is a complex condition, and this section has really only skimmed the surface. If this section has peaked your curiosity and you want to know more about this disease and its treatment, check out *Tell Me What to Eat if I Have Celiac Disease*, by Kimberly A. Tessmer, RD, LD, for more information.

Living With Digestive Disorders

After learning more about many of the most common digestive disorders, it may seem like a daunting task to live a normal life once diagnosed. But that is far from the truth. In time, you will learn more and more about managing your disease. Here are a few tips to keep in mind and to help you get started:

- Collect as much information as you can about your disease or condition. Talk to your doctor, search the Internet (making sure to stick with reputable Websites such as the ones listed in the Resource section of this book), read books and pamphlets, talk to others who have the same condition, and become aware of associations and groups that deal with your condition.

Knowledge is power, so the more you know, the more control you have over your condition.

- Educate your spouse and/or family members so they understand the basics of your condition and they can better support you.

- Don't attempt to go it alone. These types of diagnosis can sometimes be a lot to handle so seek local support groups that can add additional support and information.

- Seek the guidance of a professional when it comes to nutritional intake. Diet plays a major role in many of these conditions, and a dietitian who specializes in digestive disorders can help you sort through what is best for you and what type of diet will best control your symptoms. Contact the American Dietetic Association at *www.eatright.org* to find a dietitian in your area or ask your doctor for a referral to one.

- Make your health a priority. There will be times when your health will need to come before social activities, hobbies, work, or holidays. It can be frustrating when these things happen, but it is best to accept it and remember it won't always happen that way. There will be times that these things can take priority over your disease.

- Develop trust in others. With all the symptoms involved with IBD, it can be easy to keep it to yourself and not trust that others will understand. Many people with IBD tend to keep the knowledge of their disease to close family and friends and to try to manage most on their own. Do what is comfortable for you, but keep in mind that letting others know can make the stress of keeping it a secret much easier. Telling your boss and/or coworkers can make it easier so that they understand why you need to take time out of your day or why you might be absent from work. You may just find that people can be much more understanding and compassionate when they know what you are going through.

- Take responsibility for helping to manage your health and your disease. Those who take charge and stay involved are better able to cope than those who leave it completely up to health professionals. You can take charge by taking an active role in discussions and decisions, monitoring your changes and triggers, keeping a positive focus, and outlook and communicating with your healthcare providers.

Chapter 3

Everything You Ever Wanted to Ask a Dietitian About IBD

A part of treatment for IBD symptoms and flare-ups revolves around diet and the specific foods you eat on a daily basis. There is no evidence that any particular food or foods actually cause IBD or its inflammation, nor will they lead to remission. However, paying close attention to your diet can most certainly help to reduce some of the aggravating symptoms and can help to promote healing when your disease is active. Remember while reading this chapter that IBD can be a very individualized disease, "so there is no one diet or food fits all answer."

? What is the role of nutrition and food in IBD?

Even though there is no particular food or foods that cause or contribute to both types of IBD, experts do know that maintaining proper nutrition in managing the disease is crucial. In addition, we do know that some foods are better than others when trying to manage symptoms as well as flare-ups. Proper nutritional intake is necessary for any type of chronic disease, but especially IBD when complications such as chronic diarrhea and bleeding can rob the body of fluids and so many other essential nutrients, causing complications such as malnutrition and weight loss. Nutrition has a profound impact on our health and the proper functioning of our body's immune system. The right foods can help to boost your body's ability to fight infections and heal wounds, not to mention boost energy levels. The best thing you can do for your body is to make an effort to eat well when you are feeling well so that you are able to build up your nutritional stores for those times when you might not be feeling as well. Chapter 4 will get into more detail about which foods to include or not include during times of flare-ups and symptoms.

? What are nutritional challenges for people with IBD?

Nutritional challenges with IBD often depend on which type of IBD you suffer from, Crohn's disease or ulcerative colitis. Because Crohn's disease affects more of the small intestines where we absorb our nutrients and calories, these people run a greater risk of becoming deficient in nutrients such as vitamin D, calcium, iron, vitamin B12, and folic acid, just to name a few. In addition, because there are many foods that cause painful symptoms, it is common for these people to eat less, which leads to a lower calorie and nutritional intake. All of these factors can lead to weight loss and malnourishment. The goal is to work on getting in enough well-balanced calories to maintain nutrient needs, a healthy weight, and good bone health.

With ulcerative colitis, because it mainly affects the colon, which has a main function of absorbing water and not nutrients, the challenge is often that the patient is afraid to eat many foods because of the impact of miserable symptoms. This often leads to not consuming enough calories for adequate nutrition and ultimately weight loss. The goal for these people is getting in enough well-balanced calories and fluids in spite of an inflamed colon.

? What are the nutritional goals for IBD?

The nutritional goals for both forms of IBD involve reducing inflammation and bowel irritation through consuming nutritionally rich foods that will help to nourish the body and heal the bowel. IBD can have a significant impact on nutritional intake due to loss of appetite, inadequate food intake, increased calorie needs, especially during periods of flare-ups, poor digestion, difficulty absorbing nutrients from food and water, weight loss, and/or malnutrition. It is these types of nutritional problems that make it so important to work closely with both your doctor and a dietitian. Their goals will be to address your nutritional risk, identify your nutritional needs, and implement a nutritional plan that will help meet your individual needs to help you heal and feel better sooner.

? Is there a special diet for IBD?

There is no special "IBD diet," but there are known foods that can adversely affect the symptoms of IBD positively or negatively. Some people with IBD can tolerate just about anything when they are in remission but they have to be much more careful with their food intake when they are experiencing a flare-up, as not to add to their already-miserable symptoms. There are some people with IBD that still might experience symptoms such as diarrhea, gas, or bloating even when in remission, and food sensitivity and/or intolerance can be to blame. Eliminating problem or trigger foods can offer additional improvement for these people. Again it is important to point out that everyone with IBD will tolerate foods differently. In addition, for someone with IBD there could be additional nutritional concerns if other health problems are present, so what might work for one person with IBD might not necessarily work for another. The right diet for you is one that helps to manage your specific symptoms as well as meet your individual nutritional needs, tastes, budget, and lifestyle.

? Are there foods I should avoid if I have IBD?

Although we know that certain foods and your diet, as a whole, are not the direct cause of IBD, foods you eat can make a major difference in the severity of your symptoms, especially during flare-ups. These foods are normally termed "trigger" foods, and they can vary greatly from one person to the next. However, some foods that can commonly cause problems include dairy products, spicy foods, some high-fiber foods, and some high-fat foods. It may take some trial and error to pinpoint your trigger foods. Eliminating and then reintroducing certain foods in your diet can be a helpful technique in learning which foods you can and cannot tolerate. A dietitian can be helpful in guiding you through this process. We will dig a little deeper into this topic in Chapter 4.

? How do I know what my trigger foods are?

If you are not sure what foods may be triggering or aggravating your IBD symptoms, the best way to find out is to start by keeping a food diary for a few weeks. Play the part of the food detective by keeping a record between foods and beverages you consume as well as your eating pattern throughout the day such as when and how much you eat and their connection to your symptoms. It can also be helpful to note how you are feeling such as stressed when certain symptoms appear. The more detailed you are the easier it will be to pinpoint trigger foods and other lifestyle habits that aggravate your symptoms.

? What type of dietary guidelines can help relieve my symptoms?

There may be many factors to IBD that you cannot control, but there are plenty that you can, including diet and lifestyle. Managing your diet and lifestyle can help provide you with a sense of control, which can be a powerful motivator. We know there is no real IBD diet and not all guidelines are right for everyone. In fact, you will probably go through a bit of a trial-and-error period concerning your food intake. Pinpointing a diet plan can get frustrating at times because IBD can be changeable, and what works for a while may unexpectedly fail at other times. But stick with it, because once you get a better idea of which foods cause problems, managing your diet and symptoms should become a bit easier. Chapter 4 will provide more detail about general guidelines to follow.

? Can I just follow a healthy diet?

If you have your IBD under control and are living relatively symptom free or are in remission, there is usually no need to consume a restricted diet unless one is prescribed by your doctor for any other medical reason. At this point the prescribed diet is usually to follow a healthy, well-balanced diet. You can do that by following the USDA's (United States Department of Agriculture) Dietary Guidelines for Americans and the new MyPlate. The Dietary Guidelines for Americans are issued and updated jointly by the Department of Health and Human Services (HHS) and the Department of Agriculture (USDA) every five years. They are the guidelines that build the foundation for MyPlate, and together they work hand-in-hand. The 2010 Dietary Guidelines for Americans and MyPlate provide scientific-based advice for people 2 years and older that focus on preventing and reducing overweight and obesity through better eating and physical activity habits. The Guidelines emphasize a total diet approach by urging Americans to reduce calories by watching portion sizes; making more nutrient-rich food choices such as fruits, veggies, whole grains, and low-fat and fat-free milk and milk products; eating fewer calories from foods such as solid fats and added sugars; and by moving more. Each Guideline consists of key recommendations for various types of populations. All Americans are urged to read the Dietary Guidelines for Americans to become educated about what is recommended for a healthy diet and beneficial physical activity. The key is to adopt healthier lifestyle habits that will help to reduce your risk for numerous chronic diseases and increase your chances for a longer life. Even though you may have IBD, following a healthy diet when you are feeling well and in remission is key to staying well in all other areas of your life.

The Guidelines include specific recommendations, including:

- Balancing calories to manage weight, including maintaining appropriate calorie balance during each stage of life: childhood, adolescence, adulthood, pregnancy and breastfeeding, and older age.
- Foods and food components to reduce, such as sodium, saturated fats, dietary cholesterol, trans fats, solid fats, added sugars, refined grains, and alcohol.

- Foods and nutrients to increase, such as a variety of fruits and vegetables; whole grains; low-fat or fat-free milk and milk products; a variety of leaner protein sources (seafood, lean meats and poultry, eggs, beans, peas, soy products, nuts, and seeds); oils to replace solid fats; and foods higher in potassium, dietary fiber, calcium, and vitamin D.

- Build healthy eating patterns that meet your nutrient needs over time at an appropriate calorie level, account for all foods and beverages and assess how they are able to fit within your healthy eating pattern, and always follow food safety recommendations when preparing and eating foods to help reduce the risk for foodborne illnesses.

- Making healthier lifestyle choices, including increasing physical activity.

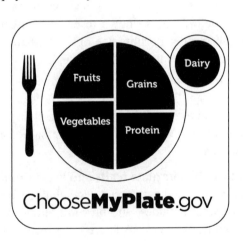

U.S. Department of Agriculture (*www.usda.gov*)
www.choosemyplate.gov/

MyPlate is a concept that helps you to take action on the Dietary Guidelines by making changes in three simple areas:

Balancing calories: Discover how many calories *you* need daily as a first step in managing your weight. Use *www. ChooseMyPlate.gov* to calculate your calorie needs. Being physically active on a regular basis can help you to balance calories.

- **Enjoy your food, but eat less.** Take the time to fully enjoy the foods you eat, but keep in mind that eating too quickly or when your attention is elsewhere can lead to eating too much and therefore too many calories. Pay attention to hunger and fullness cues before, during, and after you eat. Use those cues to recognize when to eat, how much to eat, and when you have had enough. Listen to your body!

- **Avoid oversized portions.** Use smaller plates, bowls, and glasses for your foods and beverages. Portion foods before you sit down to eat. When eating out, choose smaller portion size options, share your entrée, or take home part of your meal.

Foods to Increase: Eat more fruits, vegetables, whole grains, and fat-free or 1% milk and dairy products. These foods are full of nutrients you need for good health, including potassium, calcium, vitamin D, and fiber. Make these foods the basis for all of your meals and snacks.

- **Make half your plate fruits and vegetables.** Choose red, orange, and dark green vegetables such as tomatoes, sweet potatoes, and broccoli, along with other vegetables at meals. Add fruits to meals as part of your main dish, a side dish, or a dessert.

- **Make at least half your grains whole grains.** To eat more whole grains, simply substitute a whole-grain product for a refined product such as whole-wheat bread instead of white bread or brown rice instead of white rice. Do the same for cereals, pastas, and more.

- **Switch to fat-free or low-fat (1%) milk.** They contain the same amount of calcium and other essential nutrients as the whole version but have fewer calories and saturated or "bad" fats.

Foods to Reduce: Cut back on foods that are high in solid or saturated fats, added sugars, and salt. These can include cakes, cookies, ice cream, candy, sweetened beverages, pizza, and fatty meats like ribs, sausage, bacon, and hot dogs, and fast foods. Use these foods as occasional treats instead of everyday foods.

- **Compare sodium in foods like soup, bread, and frozen meals—and choose the foods with lower numbers.** Use the Nutrition Facts label to choose lower-sodium versions of foods such as soup, bread, and frozen meals. Select canned foods labelled "low sodium," "reduced sodium," or "no salt added."

- **Drink water instead of sugary drinks:** Cut calorie intake by drinking water or unsweetened beverages. Soft drinks, energy drinks and sports drinks can be major sources of added sugar and calories in the American diet.

The Website *www.ChooseMyPlate.gov* offers dietary recommendations, nutrition education, up-to-date information, personalized eating plans, and interactive tools as well as menus and recipes to help you plan and asses your food choices based on the Dietary Guidelines for Americans. This is the perfect place to go to put together a plan that will help balance your intake of the food groups, determine serving sizes, point out which foods are healthier to eat, estimate your daily caloric needs, and provide you with all of the general information you need to eat healthier and maintain or reach a healthy weight. For most people, that may mean losing weight, but for many people with IBD it may mean gaining weight during remission to reach a healthy weight. Following healthy guidelines can ensure you do it in a healthy manner. To check out the details of the recommendations and tools provided by the Dietary Guidelines for Americans and ChooseMyPlate, check out *www.cnpp.usda.gov/dietaryguidelines.htm* and *www.choosemyplate.gov*.

If you are in remission, don't take this time for granted. Just because your disease is under control at the present time and symptoms are not a problem, it is not a green light to go hog wild with your diet. It is the time to eat healthy and build up your nutritional stores and your strength.

Tip	The Dietary Guidelines for Americans and ChooseMyPlate are not in anyway a therapeutic diet for people with specific health conditions and may not be appropriate when your IBD is active. People with chronic health conditions such as IBD should consult with their healthcare provider and a registered dietitian to determine a dietary intake that is appropriate for them during this time.

? Is it beneficial to follow a gluten-free diet?

Because you have heard that people with celiac disease, another type of digestive disorder, must follow a gluten-free diet, you may be wondering if it may helpful with IBD as well. There is no medical indication for someone with either form of IBD to go gluten-free unless there are other known health problems indicated such as gluten intolerance or sensitivity. In fact, many foods that do contain gluten include foods that are high in fiber such as whole-grain breads, cereals, and pastas, which are great sources of fiber as well as B vitamins, and therefore can be a healthy option for someone with, for instance, Crohn's disease (when, of course, in remission). On the other hand eliminating gluten also eliminates wheat from the diet, which is one of the FODMAP carbohydrates (see the section that follows on the FODMAP approach) that for some people may cause issues. Eliminating wheat is only part of eliminating all gluten from a diet. Going gluten-free can be very complicated and can be a daunting task. It is not vital that someone with IBD follow a gluten-free diet, as it would be for someone with celiac disease. However, this has been a highly debatable topic. If you are concerned about gluten in your diet, speak with your doctor. If you want more information on celiac disease and gluten-free diets check out *Tell Me What to Eat if I Have Celiac Disease* by Kimberly A. Tessmer, RD LD.

? Can I still eat my favorite "junk" food and fast food?

It can be difficult for children and adults of all ages to think they can never have their favorite "junk" food or fast foods because of IBD. But if you plan correctly you can include some of these foods into your diet at times when you are feeling well. Take, for example, pizza, which you can make yourself and load with healthy toppings such as low-fat cheese, veggies, and lean meats. You can even sneak a hamburger or cheeseburger in there once in a while but just remember that everything should be in moderation and that these foods should be thought of as a special treat rather than a regular staple. If you adhere to the foods you know can aggravate your symptoms and you eat healthy most of the time you can enjoy a few treats now and again.

? Can I eat out with IBD?

You may have IBD but you can live a normal life, and that includes partaking in one of America's favorite pasttimes: eating out. It can sometimes be tricky, but with a little advanced planning you can have an enjoyable event. This can include a night out with friends or family, or even a business lunch. Even if you are in remission it is best to err on the side of caution and follow a few tips, because a flare-up can occur at any time. You can follow a few of these tips to make the most out of your dining out experience.

- Pick a restaurant ahead of time and do a little research on the menu before you go. Many restaurants have Websites where you can check their full menu ahead of time and know which items you will be able to eat with the least worry.

- Don't be afraid to speak up if you need something prepared a certain way. The restaurant is there to please you, so be sure to ask instead of eating something you shouldn't and suffering the consequences.

- To make you feel more at ease locate, on your own or with the help of a restaurant employee, the restrooms.

- Skip the alcohol, as this is usually not a good idea for people with IBD. Try sparkling water or a "mocktail" if you feel uncomfortable not joining in.

- Beware of appetizers such as mozzarella sticks, hot wings, and chicken fingers, which are all fat-laden and fried. All may play havoc on your digestive system. If everyone at the table is enjoying appetizers, have some bread or even a cup of soup.

? What is the best way to plan my meals?

Meal planning is a critical tool to help keep yourself well when you have IBD. Life may get busy, but you must continue to plan your meals so that you do not end up with a diet that lacks proper nutrients, which can cause all types of further problems. The best way to be sure that you will eat well for the week is to plan ahead. Think through the week and plan what you will eat for meals and snacks. From there create a shopping list and do your shopping at the start of each new week. Choose foods that you know you can tolerate from each food group, and try to eat as much of a variety as possible. Have foods on hand for those days when you are not feeling well and may have less of an appetite, as well as those days that you are feeling good and know it is a good time to stock your body with good nutrition. For most people with IBD eating smaller meals with snacks in between is the best way to get the calories, protein, and nutrients your body requires without overloading your digestive system, so when planning your meals and making your list don't forget to plan healthy snacks. Drink plenty of water throughout the day as well.

⟨?⟩ What is the FODMAPs approach?

We briefly discussed the FODMAP approach for treatment of IBS symptoms in Chapter 2, but this approach is also showing some possibility in IBD. FODMAPs may aggravate symptoms of both Crohn's disease and ulcerative colitis. As a reminder, FODMAP is an acronym for fermentable, oligosaccharides, disaccharides, monosaccharides, and polyols. FODMAPs are a group of fermentable short-chain carbohydrates that are believed to cause symptoms such as gas, bloating, and watery diarrhea in some people with digestive disorders. These FODMAP carbohydrates include lactose, fructose, fructans, sugar alcohols, and galactans (GOS). This approach looks at the total amount of these types of carbohydrates that are consumed instead of looking at each type of sugar individually.

Oligosaccharides

Fructans are chains of fructose molecules. Fructans cannot be absorbed because the small intestines cannot break them down, and this can lead to bloating, gas, and pain for some people. Wheat provides the largest amount of fructans in most people's diets. Other sources of fructans include inulin and fructo-oligosaccharide (FOS), which are commonly added to foods to increase fiber content.

Galactans (GOS) are chains of galactose molecules. Our bodies lack the enzyme to break these sugars down into digestible components, leading to gas and other GI symptoms. Galactan-rich foods include foods such as lentils, chickpeas, beans, broccoli, cabbage, Brussels sprouts, and soy-based products.

Disaccharides

Lactose is milk sugar or the sugar found in dairy products. People who are lactose intolerant have little to no presences of the enzyme lactase that breaks down lactose. This in turn causes lactose to be poorly absorbed, causing symptoms such as abdominal bloating, pain, gas, and diarrhea. This can be quite common in IBD.

Monosaccharides

Fructose is the natural sugar found in fruits. It can also be found in honey, high fructose corn syrup (HFCS), agave, and fructans. However, some fruits and fructose-containing foods will be better tolerated than others.

Polyols

Polyols are also known as sugar alcohols. They are found naturally in some fruits and vegetables, and are added to sugar-free products such as chewing gum, candy, and even some medications. They include sorbitol, xylitol, mannitol, erithrytol, and glycerol just to name a few. These polyols can create a laxative effect, causing diarrhea if a person consumes more than her or she can personally tolerate and especially when consumed along with other FODMAP foods.

The following chart will give you a better idea of what foods are included with each group of FODMAPs. The list is constantly changing as research on this data is ongoing.

FODMAPs Checklist

	LACTOSE	FRUCTOSE <0.2G/SERVING
CAUTION: HIGH FODMAPs	Milk, evaporated milk, yogurt, ice cream, custard Cheeses: ricotta, cottage, mascarpone	Fruits: apples, cherries, mangoes, pears, raspberries, watermelon Vegetables: artichokes, asparagus, sugar snap peas Sweeteners: agave, honey, high fructose corn syrup (HFCS) Alcohol: Rum
FODMAPs Friendly	Lactose free milk, lactose free ice cream, lactose free cottage cheese, lactose free yogurt and sorbet (check ingredients) Cheeses: brie, camembert, cheddar, feta, mozzrella, parmesian, swiss	Fruits: bananas, blueberries, cantaloupe, grapefruit, grapes, honeydew, kiwi, lemons, limes, passion fruit, pineapples, rhubarb, strawberries, tangelos Sweeteners: maple syrup, table sugar (sucrose) Alcohol: most wine and beer, vodka and gin (limit to 1 drink in general as gastric irritant)

Compiled by and used with permission from Kate Scarlata, RD
www.katescarlata.com/ http://katescarlata.wordpress.com

FODMAPs Checklist

FRUCTANS/GOS <0.2G EXCEPT BREAD <0.3G/SERVING	POLYOLS <0.3G/SERVING
Fruits: apples (depends on variety), nectarine, white peaches, persimmon, watermelon Vegetables: artichokes, cabbage, chickpeas, garlic, lentils, red kidney beans, baked beans, soybeans and some soymilk, onion, shallot, leeks, onion and garlic salt and powders. Grains: rye, wheat, barley (large quantities) Probiotic supplement Food additives with inulin or FOS (e.g. chicory root) Nuts: Pistachios	Fruits: apple, apricots, blackberries, nectarines, pears, peaches, plums, prunes, watermelon Vegetables: cauliflower, mushrooms, pumpkin, green pepper, snow peas. Sweeteners: sorbitol, mannitol, maltitol, isomalt, xylitol (sugar-free gum, mints, cough drops, some medications)
Tofu Vegetables: bok choy, bean sprouts, red bell pepper, lettuce, carrots, chives, spring onion (green part only), cucumbers, eggplant, green beans, tomatoes, potatoes, spinach, garlic and onion infused in oil, water chestnuts Breads/Grains: gluten free bread (check ingredients), corn, rice or quinoa pasta, rice cakes, potato and tortilla chips, rice, quinoa, oats Nuts: (10-15 max or 1-2 Tbsp.), almonds, macadamia, peanuts, pecans, pine, walnuts, pumpkin seeds, sesame seeds, sunflower seeds Moderate Fructans/GOS: limit serving size: asparagus <3 spears, beetroot <4 slices, broccoli <1/2 cup, Brussels sprouts <1/2 cup, butternut squash <1/2 cup, dried fruit <1 Tbsp., fennel bulb <1/2 cup, green peas <1/3 cup, snow peas <10 pods, sweet corn <1/2 cob	Fruits: bananas, blueberries, grapefruit, grapes, honeydew melon, kiwifruit, lemons, limes, oranges, passion fruit Sweeteners: table sugar (sucrose), glucose, maple syrup, aspartame Moderate Polyols: limit serving size: avocado <1/4, celery <1 stick, cherries <1/2 cup, lychee <5, sweet potato <1/2 cup

For this dietary approach it is a must to work with a physician and dietitian. The idea is to eliminate all foods that contain these types of carbohydrates for a trial period of around one to two weeks. If FODMAP carbs are aggravating your symptoms it would be evident by some relief of symptoms in just a few days. The next step is for the FODMAP carbs to be slowly and individually added back to the diet one at a time, to find out which ones are contributing to problems and which ones are better tolerated. The goal is to only eliminate the types of carbs that cause symptoms for that individual so that you can follow as varied and liberal of a diet as possible and not eliminate foods that are not causing problems and are not necessary to eliminate. At the end of the reintroduction phase the goal is to have a diet that only includes those FODMAP carbs that your body seems to tolerate best. Even though FODMAPs seem to have a cumulative impact, if a FODMAP is found to aggravate your symptoms, many people can still tolerate them but in smaller doses. The FODMAP approach can be complicated but if an individual is willing to try, it can be quite useful in helping to possibly manage symptoms. With any new dietary approach, it is always best to discuss it with your doctor before diving in. Keep in mind that the FODMAP approach is in its preliminary stages, especially as an approach for managing IBD symptoms.

Tip

FYI: A few FODMAP-friendly snacks might include rice cakes topped with peanut butter, cheddar cheese on rice crackers, or a handful of almonds, and an orange. You can still have a varied and yummy diet while following this type of approach.

⑦ What is the Specific Carbohydrate Diet?

The Specific Carbohydrate Diet (SCD) is a very strict, grain-free, lactose-free, and sucrose-free diet that is intended to decrease symptoms and heal people suffering from Crohn's disease and ulcerative colitis as well as celiac disease and IBS. The SCD was created by Dr. Sidney V. Haas and was popularized by author Elaine Gottschall after using it to successfully help her daughter manage ulcerative colitis. Gottschall continued research on the diet and eventually wrote a book on the topic.

Much like the FODMAPs approach, the theory behind the diet is that carbohydrates have the greatest influence on intestinal microbes (bacteria and yeast), both of which are believed to be highly involved in intestinal disorders. Most of these microbes require carbohydrates for energy. Dr. Haas believed that certain carbohydrates could promote and fuel the growth and potential overgrowth of bacteria and yeast in the intestines, and that this overgrowth could impair the enzymes that reside on the surface of the intestinal walls and keep them from functioning, which could in turn prevent the proper digestion and absorption of carbohydrates. Undigested carbohydrates in the intestines could provide even more fuel for bacteria and yeast, starting a vicious cycle. He believed that the bacteria and yeast could then form toxins and acids that could damage the lining of the small intestines and that in defense the body would produce excessive mucus to protect itself against the irritation, inflammation, and damage. According to Dr. Haas, this digestive imbalance could then develop into a number of conditions, including IBD, IBS, and celiac disease.

In light of this Dr. Haas created a diet void of complex carbohydrates that are not easily digested and instead only allows specifically selected carbohydrates that require minimal digestion, are well absorbed, and basically leave nothing for intestinal microbes to feed on, starving out the harmful bacteria and restoring balance in the gut, improving digestion. The SCD helps to correct the malabsorption, allowing nutrients to be absorbed and enter the bloodstream, making them available to awaiting cells in the body. This helps to then strengthen the system in our body that helps to fight illness, the immune system.

The lists of foods allowed and not allowed are quite extensive. The allowed carbohydrates are monosaccharides, which have a single molecular structure that enables them to be easily digested and absorbed by the walls of the small intestines. A few examples of foods allowed include natural meats (no processed meats), fish, poultry, eggs, cheese, nuts, fats, butter, and oils. Some dried beans, peanuts in the shell and natural peanut butter, are included. Non-starchy fresh and frozen vegetables and most whole fruits (no fruit juices) are allowed, as well as honey. The diet cautions to be careful of raw vegetables when diarrhea is present. Zero-carb sweeteners can be used as long as no fillers are contained. Natural cheeses such as cheddar, Colby, Swiss, havarti, and dry curd cottage cheese are allowed. Homemade yogurt is encouraged for its connection to bowel health.

Carbohydrates not allowed are disaccharides (double molecular structure) and polysaccharides (a chain of molecules). A few examples of foods not allowed include all grains such as wheat, rice, corn, oats, rice, malt, soy, buckwheat, and others. Table sugar, high fructose corn sugar, fructose, molasses, all liquid milk, canned vegetables, some beans, and legumes including soy are not allowed. You also need to avoid white potatoes, yams, margarine, some cheese (ricotta, mozzarella, cottage cheese, cream cheese, feta, and processed cheese), commercial yogurt, heavy cream, buttermilk, sour cream, and commercial mayonnaise. In addition, no bread, pasta, and other starchy foods are allowed, and the list goes on quite extensively.

The SCD can be very difficult to follow and quite restrictive, but not impossible. In fact it is several steps more restrictive than the gluten-free diet. According to the diet, strict adherence to foods allowed and not allowed is necessary to obtain any relief from symptoms. The SCD has its fans and its critics. Proponents of the diet claim quite a high recovery rate for IBD and other digestive disorders, however, critics claim there isn't enough reliable clinical trials that confirms whether it is indeed effective and which patient population it truly helps. There are plenty of true followers of the diet that believe whole-heartedly that it works. The bottom line is that if you are interested in trying this type of dietary approach it should be a topic of discussion between you, your doctor, and your dietitian. Talk with them to weigh out the pros and cons, but in the meantime be sure to keep up your current treatments.

? How can I manage my child's IBD?

IBD can show up in children. In fact, in the United States, it is estimated that as many as 100,000 kids under the age of 18 have IBD. Pediatric symptoms of IBD can include diarrhea, stomachaches, loss of appetite, weight loss, fatigue, irritability, growth issues, and unexplained fever. The best course of action is to seek treatment as soon as symptoms appear so that treatment can begin as soon as possible to help relieve symptoms. Because of its unpredictable nature it can be difficult to help your child cope with this disease and can leave the parent with a feeling of helplessness. If you are a parent you know how difficult it can be at times to get any child to eat properly, but throw in IBD and it becomes that much more important. Chronic diarrhea, poor appetite, loss of nutrients, and side effects from medications can all lead to malnutrition, which in turn can lead to growth and developmental problems.

When your child's disease is in remission or not active, the goal is to maintain a well-balanced, varied, and healthy diet that provides plenty of protein, calories, vitamins, and minerals to help them grow and develop at a normal rate. Encourage your child to

eat smaller meals throughout the day with healthy snacks in between to help manage symptoms. Have healthy foods in the house
that are readily available, and do away with the unhealthy ones so
your child won't be tempted to indulge in high-fat junk food that
can aggravate symptoms even more. Make *all* calories count by
choosing foods that your child can tolerate and that pack in the
nutrients and calories in small amounts such as peanut butter or
other nut butters, hummus, guacamole, or high-protein smoothies. Consider packing your child's lunch for school so that you
have control over what he or she are eating. Following the Dietary
Guidelines for Americans and MyPlate can again guide you to a
healthier dietary intake.

In general, there are no major restrictions to the diet of a child
with IBD unless the disease is active and symptoms warrant the
doctor to prescribe a specialized or modified diet for him or her to
follow. The type of diet will depend on the child's age and symptoms, and the area of the intestines that is being affected. During
times of flare-ups a child's appetite may decrease, the body may
need more calories to repair itself and heal and nutrients may not
be absorbed as well. The doctor may prescribe a low-fiber/low-
residue diet, lactose-free diet, and/or high-calorie diet. Additional
nutritional supplementation may also be recommended during this
time. You should work with a dietitian to guide you through any
diet modifications your child may need to follow.

It is never easy to live with a chronic illness, and kids that are
diagnosed with IBD may feel sad, nervous, and afraid. These feelings can be quite normal, and with good support most children are
able to cope with their diagnosis. However, if you find your child
is having a difficult time sleeping, eating poorly, exhibiting persistent sadness, and/or crying and showing a lack of interest in usual
hobbies or activities, be sure to contact his or her doctor. These
things can indicate that your child is having problems adjusting
and may need some additional support. Keep in mind that children
may be fatigued and may act out because they feel more irritable.

Keep an open line of communication with your child, and ensure he or she feels she or he can talk openly with his or her doctor as well. Be patient and understanding, and let your child know that you are a source of comfort and help. Let your child know that all kids are different in their own way and he or she is perfect just the way he or she is. As a parent and/or caregiver, learn all you can about IBD and talk with your child's doctor and a dietitian to help you learn to determine which foods provoke symptoms in your child and what you can do to avoid these foods. A food journal can be the perfect tool to help you in this effort. IBD is a serious condition, but with proper treatment, diet, education, and medical care, your child can live a very normal and productive life.

? Should I be concerned about nutritional deficiencies because of IBD?

Nutritional deficiencies tend to be a major concern in both types of IBD. Several factors contribute to this concern including inflammation, symptoms such as diarrhea and lack of appetite, modified diets used during flare-ups, and medications that treat IBD. Crohn's disease affects the small intestines, and that just so happens to be the spot in our bodies where we absorb the majority of our nutrients. Some of the vitamins and minerals that tend to be of concern can include iron (which can lead to anemia), calcium, folate (vital for women during childbearing age), zinc, and vitamins A, D, and K. In addition, fluid loss from diarrhea can lead to electrolyte (such as potassium and sodium) imbalances. Chapter 6 will get into more detail concerning nutritional deficiencies and IBD.

? Are there alternative nutritional supplements I can take that will help?

Many experimental treatments are currently being studied, including omega-3 fatty acids, probiotics, prebiotics, herbal remedies, and flaxseed, just to name a few. We will discuss these in more detail in Chapter 7. Always consult your doctor before considering any alternative supplements or treatments.

? Can exercise benefit IBD?

The good news is yes, exercise can definitely benefit IBD. Exercise can help reduce stress, which in turn can help decrease symptoms and possibly the frequency of IBD flare-ups. In addition, exercise can help battle some of the problems IBD sufferers encounter, including improving bone density, strengthening the immune system, increasing psychological health and decreasing depression, improving muscle strength, and combating fatigue and weight loss. Exercise can also be beneficial for those needing surgery by providing a quicker recovery, increasing stamina, preventing blood clots, increasing flexibility, and strengthening muscles after surgery.

The key, though, is to get the most out of exercise when you are feeling well. It is probably best to curtail your exercise routine during periods of flare-ups and to wait to resume it when your symptoms are under control, you are eating more regularly, your energy levels have increased, any joint pain has decreased, and you just feel better overall. If you cannot exercise you should still try to do something that can help keep stress levels down and your attitude positive, such as yoga and/or meditation. Just remember that when you are back to feeling better it is a good time to get right back to exercising. Exercise can benefit just about everyone, and that includes people with IBD. It doesn't only help to combat problems associated with IBD but your health in general.

Exercise can sometimes pose specific challenges for people with IBD, but the benefits of getting and staying in shape can typically outweigh the negatives. Here are a few tips for making exercise easier when you are dealing with IBD or any other GI disorder.

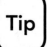 **Tip** Some medications that are used to treat symptoms of IBD may cause side effects that can make it difficult to find the energy to exercise, but don't give up the whole idea entirely. Speak with you doctor first about What might work best for you.

- Try low-impact exercises such as walking, biking, swimming, or yoga that don't require a great deal of jarring.

- If you deal with incontinence it is best to walk and not run. If using a treadmill, try increasing the elevation for more of an aerobic workout.

- Try different exercises for different lengths of time to see how your body and your gut react. Make adjustments as necessary.

- Try weight training or strength training to help rebuild muscles weakened by IBD or the medications used to treat it.

- Start slow, especially if you are not a regular exerciser, and increase your exercise intensity as you see how your body reacts.

- Listen to your body and don't push yourself physically if you don't feel up to it. Modify your routine as you need to.

- Give yourself a break when you have flare-ups or have recently been hospitalized. Allow your routine to be interrupted, and tell yourself you will get back to it as soon as you are feeling better.

- Drink plenty of water while working out. This is important for everyone but especially for those that have IBD and tend to deal with chronic diarrhea.

- Avoid eating a large meal a few hours prior to working out. Instead, try to eat small meals and snacks throughout the day.

- Most importantly let your doctor know what exercises you plan to do on a regular basis and get his or her permission first. Keep your doctors in the loop of what you are doing with your exercise routine and what changes you make.

By taking a few precautions and following some tips from your doctor, you can work exercise into your lifestyle if you have IBD. It will most definitely benefit you both physically and mentally, and will be worth the extra time and effort to do it.

Chapter 4

Tips for Dealing With Your Flare-Ups

People with IBD can go through intermittent bouts of remission. There are times they don't experience symptoms and flare-ups, and other times when symptoms can become extremely bothersome and potentially cause health concerns. This chapter will discuss diet and lifestyle habits that, for some, may cause some flare-ups or in the least aggravate symptoms when flare-ups occur. Fiber will be discussed, as this is an issue that can be confusing when you have IBD. Should I be eating a high-fiber diet or a low-fiber diet? We will also discuss special diets that are often prescribed during flare-ups that are put into place to allow the affected part of the intestines to heal.

Fighting Flare-Ups

Flare-ups for people with IBD can happen at any time. When you are experiencing a flare-up or, in other words, when your disease is active and you are experiencing symptoms, you may not feel up to eating like you normally do. By limiting some foods and choosing others that are a bit easier to digest you may help to decrease the intensity of symptoms plus get the necessary nutrition your body needs. It is best to let your doctor know when your disease is active so that both medical and dietary treatment can be prescribed if needed, and always follow your doctor's orders.

Keep in mind, as I have said over and over in this book that everyone is different regarding what foods they can and can't tolerate and what foods will and won't aggravate symptoms. No two people are the same when it comes to IBD. The suggestions in this chapter are only that: suggestions. You may have to modify your diet even more to your individual tolerance.

Foods to avoid during flare-ups

The way you eat during flare-ups may be very different from your dietary intake during remission. However, there are some general dietary guidelines of foods to avoid or limit that people with IBD can follow to help manage symptoms and improve their quality of life. It is a good idea to try to eliminate foods or beverages from your diet that seem to worsen your symptoms. As you begin to feel better you will want to check with your doctor about a good time to start easing up on your diet to include more fiber and other healthier foods that you may need to eliminate or limit during times of flare-ups. However, some of these foods may be foods you want to limit or eliminate whether you are in remission *or* experiencing a flare-up.

These are a few suggestions that may help:

- **Limit or eliminate dairy products.** If you think you may be lactose intolerant (which we will discuss later in this chapter) try to cut back on or eliminate dairy products, meaning milk and all food products made with milk, such as cheese and ice cream. People who are lactose intolerant can many times tolerate small amounts of dairy products at one time, eating dairy products as part of a meal, and/or eating yogurt. On the other hand, some people may need to eliminate lactose-containing foods altogether. If this is the case, you should speak with a dietitian who can help design a healthy eating plan that is totally void of lactose. Keep in mind that eliminating these foods will mean you need to find another source of calcium and other essential nutrients that dairy foods provide.

- **Test your fiber intake.** Though we are taught that high-fiber foods such as fresh fruits and veggies, whole grains, popcorn, nuts, seeds, and legumes are literally the heart of a healthy diet, for people with IBD these types of fiber-rich foods may cause trouble especially during flare-ups. When symptoms have subsided and you are in remission, you may be able to tolerate more fiber then when you are experiencing a flare-up. Especially during a flare-up, fiber may make symptoms such as diarrhea, abdominal pain, and gas worse. There are ways around it, such as choosing lower-fiber foods and steaming, baking, or stewing raw produce. There is also the factor of the type of fiber you consume, which we will discuss later in this chapter. Check with your doctor before you add any significant amounts of fiber to your diet.

- **Limit or eliminate gas-producing foods.** These foods might include vegetables such as broccoli, cabbage, cauliflower, Brussels sprouts, beans, onions, peppers, and carbonated beverages. Everyone is different and some foods might cause *you* more gas or less gas than others so pinpoint those foods and limit or avoid them as necessary. Keep in mind, though, that just because a few vegetables cause gas for you doesn't mean they all will.

- **Avoid greasy and/or fried foods.** These foods tend to be high in fat and are sometimes not completely absorbed by the digestive tract, which can result in the worsening of diarrhea and gas when these symptoms are present. Not to mention that greasy and/or fried foods are not part of a healthy diet whether you are in remission or in the middle of a flare-up.

- **Limit high-fat foods,** including butter, mayonnaise, margarines, dressings, and oils. Many people with IBD, especially those with Crohn's disease, have a hard time digesting fats, which can lead to worsened symptoms. You don't need to avoid them altogether but you might want to consider cutting back especially during flare-ups.

- **Avoid spicy foods,** especially during flare-ups because they can aggravate many of your symptoms.

- **Minimize salt intake.** Many times steroids are used for short-term management of flare-ups. Steroids can many times cause water retention, and consuming too much salt can further increase this symptom. To help decrease salt in your diet eat fewer processed foods and more whole foods, ditch the salt shaker, don't add extra salt to foods when you are cooking, go easy on condiments, look for "low-sodium" or "sodium-free" products, and check food labels. On the other hand, if you are experiencing frequent diarrhea and/or vomiting, you might be low in minerals such as salt and may need a more liberal intake, so check with your doctor.

- **Eat some raw fruits.** Fruit can be an important part of a healthy diet and most people with IBD do not need to eliminate all fruit from their diet. But there are precautions to take. All fruit, such as apples, should be peeled because the skins of many fruits contain insoluble fiber, which is very difficult for people with IBD to digest. For some people, skins of fruits such as peaches can be tolerated. Fruits that are fibrous, are acidic, and/or contain seeds can also cause problems, such as oranges or strawberries. If you are following a FODMAP approach be sure the fruits you choose are low in FODMAPs. Many fruits can be used in something like a smoothie to break them down and make them more easily digestible, but still watch for seeds.

- **Eat some raw vegetables.** Vegetables follow the same rule as fruits as far as some being tolerable and some not, though raw vegetables seem to pose more of a problem than fruits. They, too, are an intricate part of a healthy diet, contributing many important nutrients, so not a food group you want to completely leave out. You can include vegetables in your diet as long as you follow a few guidelines. It is best to avoid raw vegetables; cook vegetables well and peel vegetables when appropriate. Vegetables that are fibrous and contain seeds can also cause problems, so avoid those. You also want to stay away from those vegetables that are gas producing, whether they are cooked or not. Corn is a good example of a vegetable to avoid. Corn is a whole grain, and we all know from experience that corn usually comes out much the same way it goes in, so it obviously is not digested too much in the intestines. This can be too rough for an inflamed colon and/or intestinal tract.

- **Avoid red meat.** Many people find that red meat can trigger and/or aggravate their IBD symptoms. Be sure to consume enough protein but in the form of lean white meats, fish, and eggs.

- **Avoid artificial sweeteners and/or sugar substitutes.** This can include sweeteners such as sorbitol that can be found in many foods especially sugar-free foods as well as medications, so read your labels.

- **Reduce simple sugars.** This includes sweets, soft drinks, and other concentrated sugar sources. In addition to aggravating symptoms, these foods are usually high in calories but void of any real nutritional value, something your body is probably lacking during flare-ups.

- **Watch your beverages.** Avoid alcohol, caffeine, and carbonated beverages, all of which can exacerbate symptoms. Beverages that contain alcohol and/or caffeine can stimulate the intestines and make diarrhea worse. Carbonated drinks can increase the production of gas and bloating, making those symptoms you might already have feel much worse.

- **Balance your protein intake.** It is important to get plenty of protein, however, because it is difficult to stay properly hydrated, especially when experiencing a flare-up. It is best not to go too high and to divide or balance your protein intake throughout the day to avoid developing kidney stones and to give protein a better chance to be used by the body. Talk to a dietitian if you are not sure how much protein you should be getting daily, as it will depend on your individual stats.

Foods to include during flare-ups

During the active stage of IBD the goal is to eat in a way that will help to both heal and nourish your body. That might not always be easy, as some of the symptoms may leave you with an unwanted appetite. However, it is critical at this stage to get in needed nutrients and calories. Planning your diet ahead is key to providing your body with as much nourishment as you can. Some of the foods that are suggested during the active stage or during flare-ups may not seem like the healthiest of choices, such as white bread or rice, but they serve a purpose and that is to heal your GI tract while still providing your body with the energy it needs. Sticking with soft, bland foods when your condition is active will cause less irritation and discomfort. Soft foods might include hot cereals such as cream of rice; eggs; boiled, baked, or mashed potatoes; noodles; white rice; creamed soups; and streamed or cooked vegetables such as carrots (stay away from gas-producing veggies). Here are a few more suggestions of foods that you may want to consider during periods of flare-ups.

- **Low-fiber grains** such as regular white pasta, white rice, white breads, saltine crackers or Melba toast. These are complex carbohydrates that help boost your energy levels yet are low in fiber and easy on the digestive tract. These grains also pack in the calories to help maintain your weight during times of flare-ups. Toss pasta with olive oil or a healthier soft tub margarine spread and a little grated Parmesan cheese to add both flavor and calories. Mix rice with soft, cooked veggies along with fish or poultry. Try spreading smooth peanut butter or other nut butters on white bread. The key is to avoid whole grains temporarily.

- **Hot cereals** such as cream of rice or instant oatmeal can be a soothing option during a flare-up and can also provide you with complex carbs to boost energy. Choose cereals that are fortified with iron and zinc. To kick in some calories, calcium, and protein, be sure to prepare the cereal with milk. To sweeten it up a bit add some honey or a pinch of cinnamon, or even stir in some natural applesauce.

- **Cold cereals,** when choosing the right type, can actually work well during flare-ups. Now is not the time to go for the fiber-rich, whole-grain ones, though. Stick with the cereals that you are usually told not to eat such as cornflakes, puffed rice, Kix, Rice Chex, or Rice Krispies. Still, however, stick with not just the lower-fiber cereals but also the ones lower in sugar. Even though low in fiber and whole grains, these refined cereals are fortified with some much-needed nutrients such as iron and B vitamins. Use milk if you don't have a lactose problem, or mix with soy or lactose-free milk if you do.

- **Plain yogurt** can help to replenish good bacteria and promote healthy digestion. It is soothing on your GI tract and can add calcium, protein, and calories. Opt for the low-fat or non-fat yogurt and watch types with fruit that include seeds. You can use yogurt to whip up smoothies as well. Try Greek yogurt, which will double your protein intake.

- **Fatty fish**, **skinless poultry, and eggs** tend to be well tolerated during flare-ups and can boost your protein intake, which is so very important during this time of healing. Be sure to use lighter cooking methods such as grilling, baking, steaming, or broiling, and pair it with something gentle to your GI tract, such as white rice or pasta along with a steamed vegetable. When I say "fatty" fish I am of course talking about a healthy type of fat. Fatty fish such as salmon, tuna, and mackerel provide the added health benefits of omega-3 fats, which can help to ease inflammation.

- **Bananas** and other fruits easier on the digestive tract such as peeled pears, mangos, papaya, applesauce, canned peaches, or canned pears can help to provide a good source of nourishment and are generally well tolerated. You can add bananas and other tolerated fruits to plain yogurt, cereal, cottage cheese, or smoothies to boost nutritional intake and flavor.

- **Potatoes** can be a filling and nutritious food during times of flare-ups, contributing calories, complex carbs, and loads of potassium, which is a mineral that is of vital importance when it comes to maintaining the body's fluid balance. Stick to the white, fleshy part of the potato during flare-ups, as the skin is full of fiber and can cause irritation and aggravation of symptoms.

- **Soft-cooked vegetables** such as carrots, squash, pumpkin, spinach, and asparagus will add loads of healing vitamins, minerals, and phytonutrients. Soft, cooked carrots are one of those vegetables that are very well tolerated during flare-ups. You can even try juicing carrots and other vegetables for something a bit different.

- **Cheese** can help you keep up with your calcium requirements. If you have problems with lactose be sure to choose harder cheeses that are naturally lactose free or lower in lactose such as Swiss and cheddar. Avoid greasy type cheese foods like pizza or mozzarella sticks though, which will do the opposite and aggravate symptoms.

- **Other foods** might include custard, vanilla pudding, or flavored gelatin as a treat and a way to consume a few extra calories.

How to manage flare-ups

Though flare-ups with IBD will be inevitable, there are most definitely dietary and lifestyle habits that can help you to manage your flare-ups and perhaps lengthen the time between them.

- **Eliminate your problem foods.** Once you know what foods are problems for you and which ones aggravate your symptoms, make it a point to avoid these foods while your disease is in an active stage. These may include for some but not all, foods such as "gassy" foods (beans, cabbage, broccoli), high-fat/fried foods, dairy foods, high-fiber foods, raw vegetables, alcohol, caffeine, and carbonated beverages. The key is to discover what *you* can or cannot tolerate both during remission and active stages.

- **Eat smaller meals.** You may find that eating smaller meals—maybe three small meals per day with two to three healthy snacks in between, as opposed to eating three large meals—will help you feel better and ease symptoms during a flare-up and even when in remission.

- **Don't skip meals.** This can cause pain and bloating when you finally do get around to eating. Not to mention that you may be quite hungry by the time you do eat and may tend to overeat, which will, again, cause GI problems.

- **Eat slower.** Make an effort to slow down when you eat. Take small bites and chew your food well to give digestion a better chance.

- **Don't forget your fluids.** Drink plenty of fluids throughout the day, especially water. Remember to avoid alcohol, caffeine, and carbonated beverages as well as beverages high in sugar. If you suffer from chronic diarrhea you can easily become dehydrated, making you feel weak and tired. It can also affect your kidneys and lead to kidney stones, especially in warmer weather climates. If you deal with constipation, getting enough fluids can help to relieve some of your symptoms.

- **Take your vitamins.** Speak with your doctor about taking a multivitamin/mineral supplement, because IBD can interfere with your ability to absorb nutrients properly. Continue taking vitamins whether you are experiencing a flare-up or in remission. We will talk more about vitamin/minerals supplements in Chapter 6.

- **Speak with a dietitian.** If you are having problems managing your symptoms through diet, find yourself eliminating whole food groups, begin to lose weight, or just simply have questions about the best diet for you, speak with a dietitian. A registered dietitian can work with you to develop an eating plan that will help manage symptoms during acute flare-ups and help you to resume a healthy, well-balanced eating plan that will promote recovery during remission.

- **Contact your doctor.** Don't be shy about being open with your doctor about any and all symptoms you might be experiencing. It is much easier to manage flare-ups right from the start than it is to wait until it is full blown. Your medications may need to be adjusted, or you may need something added to your treatment regimen that will help. So don't suffer in silence. Never adjust your medications on your own or begin any over-the-counter medications, as that can worsen your symptoms.

Further nutritional support

If a flare-up is severe enough and there is a risk of developing malnutrition, which can greatly affect your health, a more intensive form of nutrition may need to be used. This type of nutrition support is only used if absolutely necessary. It comes in two forms: *total enteral nutrition* or TEN (tube feeding) and *total parenteral nutrition* or TPN (intravenous feeding).

TEN delivers a nutrient-rich liquid formula directly into the stomach and can act more as nutrition support rather than the only form of nutrition. Most commonly it is given through the nose and into the stomach through what's called a nasogastric or NG tube. It is most commonly given overnight and ensures that the patient receives proper nutrition. In the morning the tube is removed so the person can go about his or her everyday activities including eating if he or she is able. TEN can also be given through a gastrostomy or G-tube that is surgically inserted directly into the abdominal wall leading to the stomach. This again can be given overnight or periodically throughout the day along with eating if able.

TPN is delivered in a different method: intravenously through a catheter that is placed into a large blood vessel, usually one in the chest. It would be used as the only means of nutrition, and there would be no by-mouth feedings. This type of feeding bypasses the intestine by delivering nutrition straight into the bloodstream ,allowing the gut and bowel complete rest. TPN is sometimes required before surgery, especially if a person is very ill and cannot consume enough nutrition by mouth or by TEN. It can be used after surgery as well to allow healing. TPN can be very expensive and can create many complications, such as infection and blood clots. This method requires a specialized support team to help avoid complications and to monitor and adjust the TPN as needed.

To Fill Up or Not to Fill Up on Fiber

We have always learned that fiber is good for us and is an essential part of a healthy diet. This is true except for those with IBD who are in the midst of a flare-up. At this point some types of fiber can just be too difficult for an inflamed intestines and/or bowel to digest. In this situation consuming some foods that are too rough or raw can cause severe irritation and diarrhea. When I say "some types of fibers" I am talking about the two types of fibers: soluble and insoluble. It is basically the insoluble type of fiber that tends to cause the problem and should be avoided during flare-ups. It may help to start from the beginning to get a better understanding of what fiber is and what these two types of fibers are.

? What is fiber?

Fiber is a substance found in plants, more specifically in plant cell walls that provide plants with their shape and structure. You may also have heard of fiber being referred to as *roughage* or *bulk*. Our bodies cannot digest or absorb fiber, so it basically comes in and goes out while providing some amazing health benefits on its travels. Dietary fiber, or the fiber found in foods, is referred to as a complex carbohydrate, but because it doesn't provide nutritional value it is not considered a nutrient per se. However, you can still find it listed on food nutrient labels to help you identify foods rich in fiber.

Types of fiber

Not all fiber is created equal. Fiber is broken down into two categories: *soluble fiber* and *insoluble fiber*. They differ in their abilities to dissolve in water as well as their health effects on the body. They are both important to our health, and the key is to eat a variety of fiber-rich foods each day in order to get enough of both types of fiber. However, one is better than the other when it comes to managing IBD flare-ups. Many foods contain both types of fibers, although some may predominantly contain one type of fiber over the other.

Soluble fiber

Soluble fibers are just like they say: soluble in water. They are a fiber that soothes and regulates the digestive tract. They absorb water and form a gel-like consistency in the digestive tract, which helps slow down digestion or the movement of food in the intestines. For IBD sufferers this can help to increase the amount of nutrients absorbed and lessen diarrhea. Soluble fibers can also be helpful in producing softer stools, which can help to relieve constipation as well. In addition, these fibers don't tend to cause irritation and inflammation and can even help to relieve abdominal cramping.

Soluble fibers can pat themselves on the back for helping to lower "bad" blood cholesterol levels, which, in turn, can help reduce your risk for heart disease. In addition this type of fiber can help to slow down the rate at which glucose (or blood sugar) is absorbed by the body. This may help control blood sugar levels in people with diabetes and other blood sugar problems.

Examples of foods that contain a higher content of soluble fibers include:

- Dried beans and peas.
- Fruits (such as apricots, applesauce, bananas, apples, pears, mangoes, papayas, and grapes)—does not include the peel.
- Vegetables (such as beets, peeled potatoes, carrots, squash, pumpkin, cauliflower, and broccoli).
- Oats.
- Rice, pasta, noodles, white breads.
- Avocados.
- Psyllium seeds.

Insoluble Fiber

Whereas soluble fiber seems to be helpful for people suffering from IBD, insoluble fiber, on the other hand, needs to be consumed with a bit of caution. These types of fibers act as a very powerful GI tract stimulant, which can spell trouble for those with IBD. Insoluble fiber adds bulk to food, which helps it move along the intestinal tract, helping to avoid constipation and promote regularity. However, these fibers, unlike soluble fibers, do not dissolve in water, meaning they actually draw water into the GI tract, causing the digestive tract to move at a quicker pace. This can cause problems for people with IBD and can aggravate symptoms instead of helping them.

Limiting insoluble fibers can be tricky, though. The problem is that these fibers include a whole host of some of the healthiest foods and plenty of them. Not to mention that most foods such as grains, fruits, vegetables, nuts, and beans contain a mixture of both types of fiber. Insoluble fibers usually reside on the outside of foods and the soluble part resides on the inside for most foods. For example the skin of an apple contains insoluble fibers and the inside contains the soluble fibers.

Examples of foods that contain a higher content of insoluble fibers include:

- Whole-wheat or whole-grain breads, pasta, and cereals.
- Whole-wheat or whole-grain flours.
- Brown rice and wild rice.
- Wheat bran.
- Nuts and seeds.
- Popcorn.
- Beans and lentils.
- Fruits (such as berries, grapes, raisins, cherries, pineapple, peaches, apples with skin, oranges, prunes, melons, and grapefruits).
- Vegetables (such as spinach, kale, peas, corn, green beans, peppers, celery, onions, broccoli, cauliflower, and tomatoes).

You can't cut out all insoluble fibers, so the goal for people with IBD, especially during flare-ups, is to maintain a mixture that is more soluble than insoluble. It is best to not eat insoluble fibers alone or on an empty stomach. If you do eat foods that contain more insoluble fibers try to eat them with a food that has even more soluble fiber to try to keep a balance.

? *How much fiber should I eat?*

During a flare-up it is best to cut back on fiber and stick to soluble fibers as much as possible. However, it is also important for people with IBD to get plenty of health-promoting fiber when in remission to try to prevent flare-ups. According to the National Academy of Sciences Institute of Medicine, daily Adequate Intake (AI) for women 50 years and younger is 25 grams and 21 grams for women 51 and older. For men 50 years and younger the daily AI is 38 grams and 30 grams for men 51 years and older. Children's needs are estimated differently. A simple way to determine grams of fiber for a child older than 2 years is to add 5 to the child's age in years. For example a 5-year-old should get about 10 grams of fiber daily. After the age of 15, daily needs should be as recommended above. The key is to maintain a good combination of soluble and insoluble fibers each day to keep flare-ups at bay.

Prescribed Diets During Flare-Ups

During times of flare-ups your doctor may prescribe a special restricted diet for you to follow. This could include a low-fiber/low-roughage diet, low-residue diet, lactose-free diet, and/or even a liquid diet. This section will give you an idea of what might be included in these types of special diets. Never follow one of these types of restricted diets without it being prescribed and without being under the strict supervision of your doctor. You should also be fully instructed by a dietitian on how to follow the diet itself.

Low-fiber or low-roughage diet

A low-fiber or low-roughage diet is often prescribed for people with IBD during a flare-up or as the last step before resuming a normal diet after surgery. This type of diet is usually followed for several weeks but your doctor should instruct you specifically on the length of time you should follow the diet. This type of diet can consist of a variety of foods but emphasizes a restriction on those foods that contain the highest amounts of fiber, such as some fruits and veggies (especially those with seeds), beans, nuts, and whole grains. Eating a low-fiber diet will limit your bowel movements and is intended to help ease diarrhea and other symptoms such as abdominal pain and cramping. Once your condition is again under control, your doctor will have you slowly reintroduce more fiber back into your diet. Not following the diet as prescribed by your doctor can put you at risk for further irritation or obstruction in the GI tract. In addition, following it for longer than what your doctor prescribes can have negative effects.

The following foods would be recommended on a low-fiber diet:

- Enriched white bread.
- White rice.
- Regular plain pasta, noodles, or macaroni.
- Plain cereals that contain no more than 1 gram of dietary fiber per serving.
- Most raw, canned or cooked fruits (no seeds, membranes, or skins).
- Canned or soft cooked vegetables (no seeds, hulls, or skins).
- Well-cooked tender meats, poultry, and fish.
- Eggs.
- Smooth or creamy peanut butter.
- Dairy products such as milk, cheese, and yogurt with no seeds (unless lactose intolerant).
- Butter, mayonnaise, vegetable oils.

Tip It is usually recommended on a low-fiber diet to limit fruits and vegetables to up to two servings per day with one serving equal to ½ cup or one small whole fruit. *But* check with your doctor and/ or dietitian for specifics to your prescribed diet.

Foods usually recommended to avoid will include whole-grain breads, cereals, and pastas; brown or wild rice; dried fruits; raw fruit with skin or membranes; raw vegetables; dried beans and peas; baked beans; nuts and seeds, and foods containing them; and popcorn.

Low-residue diet

A low-residue diet is often prescribed along with a low-fiber diet during times of flare-ups or after you have had some type of abdominal surgery. *Residue* is defined as any part of food, including fiber, that remains in your GI tract, is not digested completely, and contributes to your stool output. A low-residue diet is closely related to a low-fiber diet. and sometimes the terms are used interchangeably. However, technically they are not one in the same, as a low-residue diet is a bit more restrictive than a low-fiber diet. A low-fiber diet along with a low-residue diet can help to lessen abdominal pain, cramping, and diarrhea. This type of restrictive diet may be necessary but should only be used for a short period of time, as determined by your doctor, because it can't provide all the nutrients you need long-term for good health.

The following foods would be recommended on a low-residue diet:

- Refined breads, cereals, crackers, pasta, rice. (Ideally foods should have 0 grams of dietary fiber per serving.)
- Vegetable and fruit juice with no seeds or pulp.
- Milk, yogurt (no seeds), pudding, ice cream, cream-based soups and sauces (strained). (Limit these foods to no more then 2 cups per day and avoid if lactose intolerant.)
- Strained or pureed soups made from allowed foods.
- Cooked tender meat, poultry, fish, and eggs.
- Smooth salad dressing.

- Broth-based soups (strained).

- Some canned fruits with no skin can be included as well as fruit that is peeled, cooked, and pureed. Ripe bananas are usually the only fruit that can be eaten raw.

- Butter, mayonnaise, vegetable oils.

- Foods usually recommended to avoid on a low-residue diet might include whole-grain breads, cereals, rice, and pasta; whole raw vegetables and vegetable sauces; whole fruits including canned fruits (unless otherwise specified); any foods with nuts or pieces of fruits and/ or vegetables; tough or coarse meats with gristle; peanut butter; salad dressing with seeds or pieces of fruits or vegetables; seeds and nuts; coconut; and marmalade.

This is only a general idea of a low-residue diet. It depends on your doctor and your individual case as to how restrictive your diet might be.

Lactose-free diet

People who are lactose intolerant don't make enough of the necessary enzyme lactase, found in the small intestines, to break down lactose, which is the sugar found in milk and other dairy products. When these people eat lactose-containing foods they can experience diarrhea, bloating, and abdominal cramping. These symptoms can be difficult to distinguish from the symptoms of IBD, and people who have both IBD and a lactose intolerance many times find that their symptoms worsen significantly after eating lactose-containing foods. You may be wondering why you are lactose intolerant now when you never have been. Certain health conditions, such as those of the GI tract, can create a lactase deficiency later in life, and for some people it just becomes more common as we age.

If you suspect you are having problems digesting lactose, find out for sure by speaking with your doctor. There are a few simple tests doctors can perform that will confirm lactose intolerance, such as the hydrogen breath test and the stool acidity test. There is no need to cut out all dairy products if it actually isn't lactose that is causing the problem. If you are actually lactose intolerant you need to find out just how much lactose you can comfortably consume. You need to find out how much your body can handle at one time and how many times a day your body can manage it without symptoms. Some people tolerate lactose as long as they consume the lactose-containing food with other foods and not on its own. The only way to do this is through trial and error, but it is best to know so you don't unnecessarily avoid all dairy products and their essential nutrients if you don't have to.

 Tip An intolerance to lactose is not the same thing as a milk allergy. Milk allergies are quite rare and mostly affect children who usually grow out of them by adulthood.

People have varying degrees of lactose intolerance, and some people can tolerate a little more or a little less than others. If you have a very low tolerance for lactose you may have to avoid more than just dairy products such as milk, cheeses, ice cream, and cream. You may also need to avoid any products containing whey, curds, milk byproducts, dry milk solids, and non-fat dry milk powder in addition to the obvious dairy products. There could be small amounts of lactose in breads, bread products, pastries, breakfast cereals, instant potatoes, margarine, salad dressings, cookies mixes, and the list goes on. Be sure to label read if you need to avoid lactose completely.

Food	Portion	Lactose (grams)
non-fat milk	1 cup	12.15
lactose-free milk	1 cup	0
cheddar cheese	1 ounce	.05
cottage cheese	1/2 cup	2.8
goat cheese	1 ounce	<.72
Parmesean cheese, grated	2 Tbsp.	.02
Swiss cheese	1 ounce	.02
non-fat yogurt	6 ounces	14.11 or less
ice cream	1 cup	5-7

 Tip When it somes to cheese, if the package states"zero" grams of sugar on the nutrition label then the product is lactose free, for example aged cheddar and parmesean cheese

The good news for people suffering from lactose intolerance is that there are several products on the market today that are made to be lactose free, such as some milks, ice cream, and cheeses. Soy milk, soy yogurt, and soy cheese as well as rice milk are other options because they are naturally lactose free. Many people who are lactose intolerant can tolerate yogurt without any problems, especially yogurt with live active cultures. These types of yogurts can help people digest lactose. Look for the label to make sure it states something about "contains active cultures" or "active yogurt cultures."

The biggest concern for people who are lactose intolerant is to ensure they still get enough of the nutrients found in milk products such as calcium and vitamin D. Non-dairy foods that contain calcium include dark leafy greens; broccoli; canned sardines; tuna and salmon; calcium-fortified juices and cereals; calcium-fortified soy products; and almonds. You need vitamin D to help absorb the calcium in your body. Most of us get vitamin D by being out in the sun for short periods of time, but for some who are not always in a sunny environment this can be tough. Vitamin D can also be found in fortified orange juice, fortified soy milk, fatty fish such as salmon, egg yolks, and liver. If you are not sure how to include the missing nutrients from dairy products into your diet, speak with your doctor about supplements and with a dietitian to look at alternate foods.

Liquid diets

A liquid diet is a very restrictive, very short-term diet that is mainly prescribed to provide time for the bowels to rest and heal. This may be needed after abdominal surgery or after a particularly difficult flare-up. One type of liquid diet that may be used is a clear liquid diet.

A clear liquid diet consists of clear liquids that are easily digested and leave no undigested residue in the GI tract. This diet consists of all caffeine-free clear liquids including water, tea, plain gelatin, plain popsicles, and clear broth. The next step up on a liquid diet would be a full liquid diet, which is also easily digested and easy on the GI tract. A full liquid diet is made up of fluids and foods that are normally liquid at room temperature such as ice cream. They include everything that is on a clear liquid plus juices (no pulp), ice cream (no nuts), milk, pudding, cooked refined cereal, strained cream soups, and milkshakes. Your doctor might also recommend some type of protein shake and/or high-calorie/ high-protein liquid formula as well.

If your doctor prescribes a liquid diet, you will receive specific instructions on how long to remain on the diet, and when and how to transition to a more regular diet. Never place yourself on a liquid diet without supervision from your doctor, as these types of diets do not provide enough of the essential nutrients and/or calories the body needs to function properly. Putting yourself on this type of diet for too long or too often, and not using it for what it is intended, could end up doing more harm than good by weakening the body's defenses.

Chapter 5

Tips for Managing Complications and Feeling Better

Living with IBD can create many challenges, including dealing with troublesome symptoms, health complications now and down the road, and emotional strain. The more you learn about IBD and how to manage these challenges, the more empowered you will be to live the life you deserve. This chapter will discuss some of these challenges to give you a better head start in accepting and managing them in the long term.

Managing Complications and Symptoms

IBD can involve different types of complications and symptoms for different people. You may not experience them all, but it is best to know what to expect and how to handle them if they do crop up.

Malnutrition

Good nutrition is one of the main ways the body is able to heal and restore itself to good health. Every effort needs to be made to avoid becoming malnourished, a condition that is the result of a deficiency or imbalance of nutrients in the body from lack of enough food and calories during a period of time, and diet can be an important factor. With proper nutritional status, medications tend to be more effective, the healing process is more effective, and people have more energy and feel better. Poor nutritional status or being malnourished can lead to impaired immune function, susceptibility to infections, slow wound healing, and long-term complications such as poor dental and bone health. When a person becomes malnourished, symptoms of IBD tend to become more severe and have more of a significant impact on physical and mental health.

Malnutrition can cause weight loss (or be caused by weight loss), loss of appetite, muscle weakness, and changes in skin, hair, nails, gums, eyesight, and even mood. It can be the most common reason that IBD patients end up in the hospital. Malnutrition can be caused by loss of appetite, dietary restrictions without supplementation, malabsorption of essential nutrients, medications that tend to deplete nutrient levels, infection, and/or loss of electrolytes from vomiting and/or diarrhea. If malnutrition is not corrected it can lead to a whole host of other problems and result in a vicious cycle that causes the body to improperly digest and absorb nutrients.

The best way to combat malnutrition is to eat a healthy diet to ensure you are getting all of the essential nutrients your body needs. Sounds easy enough, but this isn't always an easy feat for people with IBD. But don't worry, it will be taken step by step. The first step will be for your health team to determine if you are malnourished and to evaluate your nutritional status by checking for signs and symptoms, medical history, weight trends, diet history, lab tests, and medications. If you are showing signs of malnutrition, the next step would be for a dietitian to help manage your condition and achieve the desired health outcome by creating an appropriate nutrition plan. Your nutrition plan will be built for you and you alone, and would include individualized diet modifications and/or specialized nutrition therapies and supplementation if needed. It might even require TEN or TPN nutrition that we discussed in Chapter 4. The key is to catch any signs of malnutrition early so that your health team can work with you to get things back on track as soon as possible to avoid any short- or long-term problems.

Malabsorption

Malabsorption is a complication that can result from chronic diarrhea and/or inflammation in your GI tract and bacterial overgrowth in the small intestines, which can both decrease the absorptive surface. Less absorptive surface results in not being able to absorb enough of the nutrients from foods that the body needs for proper health and functioning. These nutrients include protein, fat, carbohydrates, vitamins, and minerals. When your body cannot absorb fat (fat malabsorption), more prominent in Crohn's disease, it can make it difficult to gain weight and especially difficult to absorb the fat-soluble vitamins A, D, E, and K. The degree to which digestion and/or absorption is impaired usually depends on how much of the small intestines surface is diseased and whether any of the intestines has been removed due to surgery. In addition, some medications for IBD can impair absorption of various vitamins and minerals.

When you are experiencing loss of appetite or even fear of certain foods such as all fruits and vegetables, which can be very common, it only compounds the problem of malabsorption. Treatment for malabsorption is much the same as it is for malnutrition including medications that help to treat the underlying problem, such as inflammation. Decreasing the inflammation or other underlying problems can help to improve intestinal absorption of nutrients. In addition, supplemental calories and nutrients are usually administered in the form of a special liquid diet. These types of supplements are made up of nutrients that are already broken down into smaller particles to allow for easier and quicker absorption into the intestines. Many times these might be administered through an enteral feeding (TEN), and if needed nutrition is given through parenteral feedings (TPN). As with the complication of malnutrition, your health team will work closely with you to get back to a point where you are absorbing the nutrients your body needs and nutrients lost have been replaced to avoid both short- and long-term health issues.

Weight loss

Many people who have IBD deal with the complication of too much weight loss, which leads to constantly trying to gain weight. This can occur due to loss of appetite or a small appetite, altered taste, chronic vomiting, fear of foods, limitations on what foods can be tolerated, malnutrition, and even from inflammation itself, which can increase metabolism. Your body may be working overtime to heal itself, which in turn can increase your calorie needs as well as nutritional needs. If you are not able to reach those basic calorie needs, weight loss and most likely malnutrition will ensue.

Keep in mind that there is a healthy way to put weight on and keep it there. Weight loss doesn't give you the green light to eat junk or get crazy with your eating habits. You still need to consider your diet as a whole and what foods you can and cannot tolerate. It may take some trial and error to see what works best for your body and what doesn't. Once you know you will be able to take necessary steps when flare-ups occur to better control your weight.

Here are a few tips to help fight weight loss and keep your weight at a healthy level. Though some of these tips may include adding certain foods to your diet, it doesn't mean that you can necessarily tolerate them.

- Eat five to six small meals throughout the day.

- Speak with your doctor about a high-calorie liquid nutritional supplement such as Ensure or Boost to supplement your diet. These are to be added to what you already eat each day and not take the place of meals to work for weight gain.

- Enjoy homemade smoothies made with foods you can tolerate (such as soy milk, almond milk, or regular milk, canned peaches, banana, or other tolerable fruits, flax seed, protein powder, wheat germ, and/or yogurt).

- Use smooth nut butters on bread, toast, or crackers, such as almond, peanut, cashew, or soy nut butter, for a good dose of calories, protein, and healthy fats. A small amount delivers a ton of calories.

- Try ripe avocados, which are very high in calories and healthy fats. You can eat them plain, sliced on sandwiches, pureed as a spread, pureed in a smoothie, or as guacamole dip.

- Add hummus to your diet on pita bread, as a spread for sandwiches or burgers, or as a dip.

- Add olive oil or a healthy margarine spread to foods such as vegetables, eggs, and mashed potatoes, or to any of the dishes you make to add a boost of calories. You can even add a bit of oil to your smoothies to add extra calories. Extra-virgin olive oil is very heart healthy.

- If you are trying to gain weight avoid too much high-intensity aerobic exercise because it tends to burn so many calories. Don't stop exercising, but consider sticking with light or brisk walking or light strength training to help you maintain and even build some muscle mass. Always be sure you are eating enough to cover the extra calories burned and then some.

- If you can't seem to gain weight no matter what your efforts, speak with your doctor and a dietitian.

> **Tip**
>
> FYI: Not everyone with IBD has the problem of weight loss. Certain medications such as prednisone, which is a common medication used in IBD, can cause weight gain. The weight gain is typically due to fluid retention, increased appetite, and fatigue leading to decreased physical activity, all side effects from the medication. Most side effects are reversed once the dosage is decreased or stopped. However, even if you are gaining weight never stop your medication without speaking with your doctor.

Loss of appetite

Staying well-nourished can be a difficult task for people with IBD who are experiencing a flare-up. During a flare-up eating enough calories, protein, and other nutrients to meet your needs doesn't always seem possible. People tend to lose their appetite due to symptoms such as pain, nausea, fatigue, and diarrhea. Loss of appetite can lead to weight loss and malnutrition. Be sure to speak with your doctor if you can't manage to eat much. Try to think of foods that stimulate your appetite, make sure you eat when you feel good enough to, and make those calories count. Follow some of the previous tips for gaining weight.

Constipation or diarrhea

Constipation and persistent diarrhea can both be symptoms that people with IBD deal with, though diarrhea is much more common. One main concern with frequent diarrhea is the loss of electrolytes and occurrence of dehydration. Signs of dehydration can include dry mouth, excessive thirst, dry eyes, and infrequent urination. The extent of diarrhea can be dependent on location, extent, and severity of inflammation in the GI tract; malabsorption; altered motility; medications, and/or diet. Persistent diarrhea is usually treated with medication therapy, but because not everyone with IBD has the same extent of diarrhea, it is essential for your therapy to be tailored to your individual condition. As for constipation in IBD, it is usually present due to a bowel obstruction and slowed transit. Chronic constipation can cause additional problems so let your doctor know if this symptoms occurs. Your doctor may prescribe some type of laxative and/or fiber supplement, depending on your individual case. In both cases (of either diarrhea or constipation) it is essential to drink plenty of water.

Cramping, bloating, and/or gas

One chief complaint from people who have IBD is abdominal cramping, bloating, and gas. For people with IBD, the process of digesting food can bring on symptoms of cramping, bloating, and gas, as well as some of the other symptoms we discussed such as diarrhea. Bloating and some abdominal cramping can at times largely be caused by intestinal gas. What brings on the gas? It can be caused by eating gassy foods or foods that your GI tract cannot tolerate, swallowing air while eating, drinking carbonated beverages, and/or lactose intolerance. Getting too much fiber in the form of insoluble fibers can also cause problems of gas, bloating, and abdominal pain for people with IBD.

Tip There can be more serious reasons for bloating other than gas. If your abdomen is tender to the touch or feels hard, be sure to contact your doctor. Persistent, progressive, and severe bloating that is accompanied by other symptoms should not be taken lightly and should be checked out by your doctor immediately.

These can all be very uncomfortable symptoms, but there are ways to try to deal with them. Try to slow down when you eat, eat smaller meals, don't talk while you are eating, avoid greasy and fried foods, and limit milk and dairy products if you suspect or know you are lactose intolerant. Also avoid foods that you know cause you gas as well as foods that generally cause gas for most people such as broccoli, cabbage, cauliflower, corn, and asparagus. In addition, get plenty of exercise, if you are able, to keep your intestines moving properly. Your doctor may prescribe medications to help with some of these symptoms as well.

Tip

Never take over-the-counter medications for any symptoms such as diarrhea, gas, or constipation without first speaking with your doctor. Sometimes they can do more harm than good.

Food fears

Food fears are all too real for people with IBD. If you have lived with an obstruction, stricture, or other serious complications that has caused relentless symptoms and strict dietary changes, it can be daunting to try certain foods again even after surgery has removed the obstruction or you are in remission. Certain foods for you can leave painful memories. The motivation to avoid pain at all cost and stay away from any questionable foods can be a strong one. It can be quite normal to feel apprehensive about eating a more normal diet again. Taking it slowly and adding new foods one at a time as you feel comfortable can help. Remember to chew food thoroughly, eat slowly, and eat smaller portions. The goal is to facilitate a good relationship with food and eating even after it has caused so many problems in the past. The restricted diets you have been on should be reassessed frequently so they can be adjusted and as regular a diet as possible resumed. If foods continue to give you problems, eliminate them if necessary, but the idea is to try them so you are not following a restricted diet for a lifetime if you don't have to. A dietitian can help you to feel comfortable about adding foods back into your diet, and can help guide you slowly and carefully through the process.

Decreased bone density

People with IBD, especially Crohn's disease, are at a greater risk for having decreased bone density due to malabsorption, decreased appetite, lactose intolerance, and steroid medications. All of these can create a loss of calcium and vitamin D absorption, and therefore increase bone loss and jeopardize the stability of healthy bones. In addition, Crohn's disease itself has been shown to possibly be linked to osteoporosis. Bone loss can lead to most importantly osteoporosis later in life. Osteoporosis is a bone disease that causes thinning of the bone tissue and loss of bone density. It can cause compression fractures of the spine, disability caused by very weak bones, and wrist and hip fractures.

To combat this problem it is essential to get an ample amount of calcium and vitamin D, a fat-soluble vitamin that promotes calcium absorption. According to the Food and Board (FNB) at the Institute of Medicine of the National Academies, adults ages 19 to 50 years of age should aim for at least 1,000 milligrams (mg) of calcium daily. Adult women 51 to 70 years need at least 1,200 mg daily, and men in this age range need 1,000 mg. Adults 71 years and older need to shoot for 1,200 mg. You can get too much of a good thing, usually from excessive supplement use, and the FNB warns that the Upper Tolerable Limit for calcium is 2,500 mg for adults 19 to 50 years and 2,000 mg for adults 51 years and older. Your best bet is to get your calcium from a combination of food and supplements that are divided into three doses throughout the day for optimum absorption. According to the FNB, most adults ages 19 to 70 years should shoot for about 600 IUs (international units) of vitamin D daily, though most experts feel that should be more. For adults older than 70 years the goal is 800 IUs. The Upper Tolerable Limit for vitamin D is 4,000 IUs. Speak with your doctor about types and amounts of supplements that will work best for you.

Tip For recommendations on children younger than 19 years, check out the Dietary Guidelines or ask their pediatrician. Food and Nutrition Information Center: *http://fnic.nal.usda.gov*

If you can handle dairy then you are in luck, because these foods are chock full of calcium and vitamin D, especially milk. If you are lactose intolerant you can still find alternate substitutions that will supply these nutrients such as soy milk, almond milk, rice milk, lactose-free milk, and soy yogurt. All are great substitutions for cow's milk with comparable amounts of calcium and vitamin D. Be sure to read the food label, though, to make sure you are getting what you think you are.

Speak with your doctor about being screened for bone density if you are at risk. The earlier signs of decreased bone density are caught the more time there is to implement preventable treatments.

Joint pain

IBD can literally be a pain in your neck, or more common, your elbows, wrists, knees and/or ankles. It is estimated that about one in four people with IBD, especially Crohn's disease, will develop some type of arthritis or inflammation of these joints. Although IBD is a disease of the digestive tract, it can manifest as inflammation in the joints as well. For most people the pain usually comes and goes and shows up in different joints in the body, so it is known as migratory arthritis. Most of the time once the symptoms of IBD have been treated or a person is in remission the joint pain will leave as well with no permanent damage to the joints.

Let your doctor know if you experience joint pain, as there are medications that can help to relieve your pain. Staying physically active can help if you are able and your doctor allows it. Drink plenty of water as well, which can help lubricate joints and help keep the swelling down. Omega-3 fatty acids can also be helpful as a natural inflammatory, but speak with your doctor before taking any supplements.

Lifestyle Changes That Count

You may feel helpless as you deal with your IBD, but the good news is there are lifestyle changes you can make, in addition to diet, that can count in a big way to help reduce and relieve some of your symptoms. Making positive changes in your life can help you to feel empowered when it comes to dealing with your disease and help you to realize that what you do can make a difference!

Reducing your stress levels

Managing stress in your life is something we all need to strive for but it is extra important for people with IBD. Stress may not cause IBD, but it sure can play a role in aggravating symptoms. Stress has a tendency to increase blood flow to our GI tract. This in turn increases motility and stimulates contractions in the intestines, which can lead to symptoms such as diarrhea and nausea. For people with IBD, who are already susceptible to these types of GI symptoms, stress can make them that much worse. Experts also believe that stress can increase inflammation and stimulate flare-ups of IBD.

For people with IBD, being able to manage everyday stressors not only helps with physical symptom management but emotional symptoms as well. Managing stress can help decrease your risk of feeling depressed and/or anxious. This can most definitely make living with IBD much more manageable.

There are steps you can take to help reduce your stress:

- Seek out emotional support from family and friends. Have a support system that you know you can lean on at times when you are not feeling your best.

- Seek out emotional support from IBD support groups and others who deal with your same situation. There are many support groups both on-line and locally in your area that can be helpful to you with suggestions on how to manage and live with your disease and offer emotional support. Only people that are going through your same situation can honestly know how you are feeling and that can be a big support. Check the Resource Guide.

- Consider seeking out professional help from a psychiatrist or psychologist, especially if you are dealing with depression and/or anxiety. Dealing with IBD or other chronic illnesses is difficult and seeking out help is most certainly nothing to be ashamed of. Do not suffer in silence!

- Stress can often cause sleep disturbances and fatigue. Fatigue can then affect the immune system, which can then possibly cause IBD flare-ups. Try your best to get sufficient sleep at night and rest throughout the day if needed. If you are having trouble sleeping, don't let it go, speak with your doctor.

- Try to be physically active as much as possible. It may be difficult at times, but regular exercise can help to relieve stress, relieve anxiety and depression, help you sleep better, help fight fatigue, and help you to feel better in general. Doing something is better than nothing at all, so do your best to try to be active every day. Check with your doctor before starting any type of exercise program.

- Try yoga, which is very holistic, meaning it combines mind and body. Yoga can be a great stress reliever and has quite a calming effect. For purposes of stress relief and healing choose a type of yoga that is gentle and focuses on meditation. Check with your local gym or recreation center to find a certified instructor who specializes in areas of stress relief as well as digestion.

- Try other forms of stress-reduction therapies such as Reiki, meditation, or acupuncture. We will discuss these in more detail in Chapter 7.

- Put aside time every day for *you* to do activities that help you relax. Do what you find relaxing, such as reading, listening to music, walking, taking a warm bath, talking with a friend, and so on.

Kick the smoking habit

If you are a smoker and have IBD, you have another reason to kick the habit. Smoking has numerous related health risks that we all know about, and you can add to that being detrimental to IBD suffers, especially those who have Crohn's disease. In fact, smoking can make the disease more aggressive and may even increase one's risk for contracting it in the first place. Crohn's disease tends to come back more quickly and with more vengeance after surgery in smokers. In addition, those with Crohn's who continue to smoke are less likely to respond to medical therapy. One theory seems to be that because smoking causes constriction of the blood vessels, it can lead to an inadequate flow of oxygen and nutrition to the intestines, causing harm to the area.

On the other hand, for reasons still unknown, it is actually non-smoking that seems to be associated with the incidence of ulcerative colitis, and there is evidence that smoking cigarettes may improve the disease severity and even have a protective effect in some people. However, the mechanism that creates this association between smoking and both Crohn's disease and ulcerative colitis is not known at this time. So keep in mind that this does not imply that smoking would improve symptoms of ulcerative colitis. At this point the hefty health risks of smoking definitely outweigh the possible benefits. Your best bet, no matter which type of IBD you suffer from, is to stop smoking and find a healthier way to relieve stress and tension! If you need help kicking the habit, speak with your doctor.

Get your body moving

Exercising might be the last thing on your mind when you have IBD, but it can truly help you to feel better both mentally and physically. Aside from the basic benefits that exercise provides the general population such as improved cardiovascular health and maintenance of a healthy weight, physical activity for those with IBD can help to decrease stress, increase circulation, boost energy levels, induce feelings of well-being, increase self-esteem, improve muscle tone, strengthen bones, reduce the risk for developing colon cancer, reduce depression and anxiety, help maintain a healthy body weight, and aid digestion. In fact, a few studies have shown that for people with IBD, mild exercise, such as walking just 30 minutes three times per week, can in general decrease disease activity and symptoms. The key is to find something you enjoy, and not to think of it as exercise but as a regular activity. Start slow at whatever activity you choose and increase slowly. Remember that as long as you are doing something to move your body, it is better than nothing!

You may have to test your body's limits and see which exercises fit you best. For some people high-intensity workouts such as aerobics or running can be tough on the GI tract and have you running to the bathroom more then you care to. To avoid this, try lower-impact activities that are a bit easier on your body such as walking, biking, or swimming. See what fits you best and do it on a regular basis to see benefits. Regardless of which form of exercise you choose, always check with your doctor first and keep him or her in the loop, especially if you notice any change in your IBD symptoms. Remember to keep your body well hydrated when you are exercising.

> **Tip**
>
> During a flare-up take it easy on the workouts. Your body is already working hard to fight your IBD symptoms, so don't push yourself and make your body work overtime. However, don't stop exercising! Just use gentler exercises, unless your doctor tells you otherwise, at the time of flare-ups, such as yoga, swimming, light weights, or walking, and save the rigorous exercise for times between flare-ups when you are feeling better.

Learn to cook

If you have IBD you know how difficult it can be sometimes to eat out on a regular basis or to eat processed foods that contain "safe" ingredients. Your best bet is to cook for yourself; if you don't know how, learn. Learning how to prepare safe, healthy, and delicious meals can be an invaluable skill to someone with IBD. Maybe you already know how to cook but it is a matter of taking the time to do it. Invest in some new cookbooks, or take a class if cooking isn't your forte or you need a bit of motivation. Swapping recipes with friends can be a fun way to try some new dishes and can make it fun. If you belong to an IBD support group a recipe swap can be a great event! Check out chapter 8 for some great recipes. In addition Chapter 9 lists some terrific cookbooks and websites that offer delicious recipes. Bottom line is that it can make living with IBD much easier and less stressful, can boost your overall nutritional intake plus save you lots of money!

Deal with depression and anxiety

Like many other serious chronic illnesses, IBD can ultimately lead to depression and anxiety. It can be a vicious cycle as the disease can cause a certain amount of depression and anxiety to occur, and in turn both of these can worsen symptoms and impair recovery, which in turn can cause depression and anxiety to increase. The key is to be able to recognize that you are feeling depressed and/or feel anxious so that you can take the necessary steps to get them under control before they take control. Signs that you could be dealing with depression and anxiety might include:

- Persistent sad and/or anxious mood.
- Loss of interest in activities you once enjoyed.
- Lack of interest in engaging socially with others.
- Changes in appetite or weight loss that don't seem to be related to your disease.
- Trouble sleeping or sleeping too much.
- Trouble concentrating, remembering, and/or focusing.
- Irritability, agitation, and/or restlessness.
- Fatigue and feeling of decreased energy.
- Thoughts of death or suicide.

Most importantly, if you feel you have any of these symptoms and are not quite sure whether you are dealing with depression and anxiety or not, speak with your doctor. Everyone can get down in the dumps from time to time, but for people with chronic illnesses such as IBD it can be quite common for a case of the blues to last a bit longer. Never be ashamed to speak up, as treating depression and anxiety is important to your overall health. A positive mental outlook is imperative to your health and well-being, and can help you recover quicker from flare-ups or surgeries.

An initial diagnosis of IBD can be tough so give yourself plenty of time to deal with your feelings, but then try to move on with your life, get involved in activities you enjoy that have nothing to do with IBD, be honest with your friends and family and create a strong support system, take care of yourself physically by getting plenty of sleep, eating healthy, stopping smoking if it applies to you, avoiding alcohol, exercising regularly, and practicing relaxation techniques. Even when you are feeling down and it seems like your symptoms will never end, remember that they will and that you will not always feel this way, and never be tempted to stop any of your mediations or make any changes on your own.

The Benefits of a Food Diary

People keep food diaries for all different types of reasons. They may keep them to lose weight, improve health, keep track of food allergies or sensitivities, or keep note of what foods may be causing certain symptoms. A food diary is basically a detailed record of what you have eaten or drank over a certain period of time. If you have IBD you may be asked by your doctor and/or dietitian to keep a food diary or it may be something you want to get started with on your own.

Why keep a food diary?

I have mentioned numerous times that everyone with IBD is different when it comes to the foods that will and won't aggravate their symptoms, especially during a flare-up. There is most definitely a list of general foods that for most should be avoided during a flare-up. However, that, too, will differ for individuals and the key is to avoid only the foods you need to and nothing more. No need to keep entire food groups or foods out of your diet if they are not causing you problems! Keeping track of the foods and beverages you consume each day along with your symptoms can be a very valuable tool in helping to identify the offenders or foods that may trigger *your* symptoms. Avoiding these foods, especially during a flare-up can give you better control of symptoms, and that is the goal.

 Tip If writing your food diary in a notebook isn't your thing try, keeping track on your computer. Keep your eye out for apps that may come out for your phone as well, which can help make keeping a food diary even more convenient.

Not only can a food diary help you to identify your individual trigger foods, but it can also help your doctor and dietitian to determine whether you are getting enough of all the essential nutrients your body needs to heal and be in good health, such as protein, carbohydrates, fats, vitamins, and minerals. In addition it can clue them in to whether or not you are getting enough calories to maintain a healthy weight as well as your energy levels.

How best to keep a food diary

Keeping a food diary can be simple as long you as keep up with it. All you need to do is record the foods you eat and beverages you drink throughout the day. Remember that everything you put in your mouth counts! It is helpful to note approximate serving sizes as well. Enter the date, meal or time, food and/or beverage, serving, size and any symptoms you might feel after eating the food and/or beverage. It is easiest to jot down the foods, beverages, and symptoms in your journal as soon as you consume them. Waiting until the end of the day will take you more time, and you may forget foods you ate throughout the day or forget how you felt by the end of the day, which won't do you much good. However, if time doesn't permit during the day then be sure to take some time at the end of the day to carefully think through your day and jot down everything you can recall. The more specific you are, the easier it will be to pinpoint trigger foods and the better your doctor and/or dietitian will be able to determine whether you are getting all the nutrients you need. Don't worry, you won't need to keep a food diary forever! But you will need to keep one long enough to be able to supply the information your doctor and dietitian need.

After a set amount of time, set up an appointment to review your food diary with a dietitian so that he or she can help you to pinpoint your trigger foods and analyze your nutritional intake. The dietitian can make necessary change to your diet as needed to ensure it is well balanced, contains sufficient calories to keep you at a healthy weight, and is free of your problem foods.

Follow these easy steps to start your food diary:

- Get a notebook that is small enough to carry with you.
- Use a new page for each new day, and organize each page into columns.
- Use the first four columns for what you ate or drank, the serving size, where you ate, and what time you ate. Be very specific and don't forget things like condiments added to sandwiches, creamer added to coffee, or dressing added to salad.
- Use a column for noting *any* symptoms (such as diarrhea, gas, bloating, cramping, and so on) that you experience and the time they occurred. Keep in mind that some symptoms won't show up right away.
- Include a column for your mood as well as energy level. Note if you were stressed or upset when you ate.
- If your food diary is going to work to your benefit, you need to honest and thorough about everything you eat and drink throughout the day, even if you sneak a few cookies at 2 a.m. No one is using your diary to judge you, just to help you!

Sample food diary

		My IBD Food Diary Date: _____				
Time	Where I Am Eating	Food/Drink Consumed	Serving Size	Symptoms/ Severity	Time Symptoms Occured	Stress/ Feelings/ Energy Level

Chapter 6
Supplementing Your Diet

A properly balanced diet is chock full of all the essential nutrients our bodies need for good health and proper functioning. When we don't get enough of certain nutrients such as vitamins and minerals to promote good health, it is known as a nutrient deficiency. People with IBD are at greater risk for nutritional deficiencies. This chapter will discuss why people with IBD are at greater risk and will discuss in detail some of the more common vitamins and minerals that can become a problem.

The Need for Vitamins and Minerals

Individuals with IBD, especially those with Crohn's disease, are at a greater risk for nutritional deficiencies for a whole host of reasons. For those with Crohn's disease, inflammation of the small intestines creates a problem because this is where the majority of fat, protein, carbohydrate, and absorption of vitamins and minerals takes place. This can lead to deficiencies of water-soluble vitamins including many B vitamins and most of the fat-soluble vitamins. For those with ulcerative colitis, where inflammation takes place in the large intestines, the problem is the decreased absorption of electrolytes such as potassium, water, and the production of vitamin K. Diarrhea in ulcerative colitis can also lead to folic acid, calcium, and other electrolyte deficiencies. In addition to these problems is loss of appetite due to nausea, vomiting, or stomach pains; consuming a very limited diet; and/or medications used to treat IBD that can cause some deficiency problems.

The way in which the body uses and absorbs vitamins and minerals is an integrated and complex one. Many nutrients need the presence of other nutrients to facilitate their absorption and be used by the body. If the body is short on just one vitamin, the end result can be a chain reaction that affects the absorption and use of many other vitamins and minerals. It is important to understand what some of these vitamins and minerals do for our body and why a deficiency can be harmful.

Vital vitamins

Vitamins may be in the "micronutrient" category, but they are far from "micro." Vitamins are organic compounds and a group of nutrients that are very powerful but required in small, even tiny, amounts to do their very important jobs. Vitamins are involved in just about every function in the human body, from the digestion of food to the regulation of body processes. The problem when diet is limited, absorption from food is impaired, and food intake is decreased is that most of the vitamins our body needs come from the foods we eat. There are 13 essential vitamins that our body needs to function properly, and these vitamins are divided into two groups called water-soluble and fat-soluble vitamins. Their descriptive names explain how they are both carried in food and transported in the body.

Fat-soluble vitamins

Fat-soluble vitamins consist of vitamins A, D, E, and K, though it is vitamins A, D, and K that pose the most deficiency problems for those with IBD. These vitamins dissolve in fat, and that is how they are carried throughout the bloodstream and the body. This is one reason we need some fat in our diets. It is also a reason why those people with Crohn's disease who deal with fat malabsorption (have a hard time absorbing fat) have a risk of becoming deficient in these types of vitamins. Fat-soluble vitamins can be stored in fat tissue and the liver, so it can be detrimental to consume excessive amounts of these vitamins, especially in the form of supplements, over a long period of time.

> **Tip**
>
> Contrary to popular belief, vitamins do not directly supply energy because they do not contain calories. However, they do regulate and are needed for the breakdown or metabolism of fats, proteins, and carbohydrates that *do* directly supply energy or calories to the body.

Vitamin A

Vitamin A deficiencies are not all that common, but they can occur in someone with IBD, especially those with Crohn's disease who, because of inflammation, cannot absorb enough of this vitamin in the small intestines. In addition, adequate protein levels are needed to carry vitamin A that is stored in the liver into the bloodstream, so for those with protein calorie malnutrition even supplements may not raise vitamin A levels without adequate protein. Another reason to get plenty of protein!

You may have heard growing up that eating lots of carrots will help you see well. Well, that is pretty close to the truth because carrots are full of beta-carotene, a powerful antioxidant that is known as pro-vitamin A, and can be converted into vitamin A in the body. Carotenoids, such as beta-carotene (considered the most important of the pro-vitamins), are found only in plant foods. The body can use them to synthesize vitamin A according to need and, therefore, in people with IBD a high intake of beta-carotene is important. Carotenoids, unlike pre-formed vitamin A, are non-toxic in any amount. Preformed vitamin A supplements can be toxic to the body as well as cause birth defects in doses that are too high, so speak to your doctor before taking a vitamin A supplement.

Body basics

Vitamin A plays an essential role in promoting normal vision, growth, health of body cells and tissue, cell reproduction, maintenance of healthy hair and skin, and regulating our immune system to help fight off infection. A deficiency of vitamin A can lead to night blindness and a diminished ability to fight infections. The Dietary Reference Intake (DRI) for vitamin A is 700 micrograms (mcg) for adult females and 900 mcg for adult males. However, those with IBD who are at risk for vitamin A deficiency may need more. The Upper Tolerable Limit to be aware of is 3,000 mcg.

Best food sources

Pre-formed vitamin A can be found in liver, milk, fortified breakfast cereals, and eggs. Pro-vitamin A such as beta-carotene can be found in orange, red, yellow, and dark green veggies, and fruits such as carrots, cantaloupe, spinach, sweet potatoes, and mango.

Vitamin D

People with IBD can lack vitamin D due to poor absorption, not receiving much sun exposure, and/or not having enough calcium, which the body needs to properly use vitamin D. People with IBD, especially Crohn's disease, tend to poorly absorb fat-soluble vitamins such as vitamin D because fat is poorly absorbed when there is active inflammation in the small intestines. In addition, certain medications taken for IBD such as prednisone can interfere with calcium absorption, decreasing the body's ability to properly utilize vitamin D.

Body basics

Vitamin D is important to the absorption of calcium and phosphorus, and for depositing them in the bones and teeth to help make them strong. Vitamin D is also responsible for the regulation of cell growth and for protecting the immune system. A deficiency of vitamin D can lead to osteomalacia or soft bones in adults, which can make you susceptible to bone fractures. In children a deficiency can lead to rickets, which also leads to softening of the bones and skeletal deformities. The DRI for vitamin D for adults up to 70 years of age is 600 international units (IUs) and 800 IUs for adults older than 70. Just as with vitamin A, those with IBD may need a different amount. Too much vitamin D can also have detrimental health effects. The Upper Tolerable Limit to be aware of for adults is 4,000 IUs.

Tip Discuss vitamin D supplements with your doctor as they have the potential to interact with several types of medications including steroids.

Best food sources

Vitamin D is best known as the "sunshine vitamin" because believe it or not we can get vitamin D from the sun. Vitamin D is actually synthesized by the body when our skin is exposed to moderate amounts of sunlight for short periods of time. You don't need a ton, so don't use that as an excuse to spends hours in the sun with no protection! Luckily for people who don't get much sun exposure, there are also foods that supply vitamin D, including fortified milk, yogurt, juices, and margarine; eggs; fish liver oils such as cod liver oil; fatty fish (salmon, canned sardines, tuna, and mackerel); some fortified cereals; and liver. Because many people with IBD are also lactose intolerant and avoid dairy products, paying attention to fortified foods, taking a calcium supplement with vitamin D, and getting a bit of sun exposure may be needed.

Whether you are getting vitamin D from the sun and/or from foods, it is usually still poorly absorbed by those with IBD, especially Crohn's disease, so speak to your doctor about possible supplementation in order to maintain proper levels of vitamin D. Regular monitoring may also be needed in order to ensure your levels are staying steady.

Vitamin K

People with IBD, especially those with Crohn's disease, can become deficient in or have low levels of vitamin K due to poor food intake as well as poor absorption by the small intestines. In many studies it has been found that blood levels of vitamin K were significantly reduced in people with IBD.

Body basics

Vitamin K aids the body in the regulation of blood clotting to help stop bleeding. It also helps in the production of a special protein that is essential for helping calcium bind to bones. Although for most people, a vitamin K deficiency is rather rare, people with IBD are at a definite risk because they have problems absorbing fat-soluble vitamins. Not getting enough or having low levels in the body can result in more bruising and bleeding. A deficiency of vitamin K along with a deficiency of vitamin D often contributes to the bone density loss found in people with IBD. A vitamin K deficiency can also occur due to long-term antibiotic use, which can lessen its absorption, and from chronic diarrhea.

The DRI for vitamin K for adult females is 90 mcg and for adult males is 120 mcg. Just like with other fat-soluble vitamins, the amount of vitamin you may need if you have IBD may be different than those of the established DRIs. No Upper Tolerable

Limit has been set for vitamin K at this time. However, it can be toxic at very high levels, so speak with your doctor about a supplement dosage that is right for you.

 Tip If you take a blood thinner such as warfarin (coumadin) keep in mind that vitamin K and foods containing vitamin K can affect how the drug works. Speak with your doctor concerning how much vitamin K is safe for you to take.

Vitamin K is a little different from other vitamins in that it is actually made inside the body by "good" bacteria in the large intestines or colon. In a healthy GI tract, about 80 percent of the vitamin K our body needs is made this way, with the other 20 percent coming from food sources. For people with IBD, that "good" bacteria in the intestines can be wiped out by antibiotics as well as chronic diarrhea, which can diminish vitamin K production in the body.

Best food sources

As far as food sources, vitamin K can be found in green leafy vegetables such as kale and spinach, and other veggies such as green beans, Brussels sprouts, asparagus, cabbage, cauliflower, broccoli, peas, and carrots. If these veggies sound familiar that is because they are usually ones that people with IBD need to or want to stay away from. Vitamin K can also be found in some legumes such as soybeans and black-eyed peas, some nuts, and some fortified cereals.

Water-soluble vitamins

Water-soluble vitamins dissolve in water and are carried through the body by watery fluids. Unlike fat-soluble vitamins, most water-soluble vitamins are not stored in the body, at least not in significant amounts. The body uses what it needs when it comes to these vitamins, and the remainder is excreted through the urine. Because our bodies don't store these vitamins we need a constant supply from the foods we eat to ensure our bodies have optimal amounts. There is less of a worry with toxicity when it comes to water-soluble vitamins, but more worry when it comes to deficiencies. The water-soluble vitamins consist of eight B vitamins: thiamin (B1), riboflavin (B2), niacin (B3), pyridoxine (B6), cobalamin (B12), folate, pantothenic acid, biotin, and vitamin C. We will discuss a few of these water-soluble vitamins that are of most concern for those with IBD.

Vitamin C

Vitamin C is also known as ascorbic acid and besides its job as a water-soluble vitamin, it also acts as a powerful antioxidant. A deficiency of vitamin C, which causes scurvy, is rarely seen. But it is important to mention this vitamin because people with IBD tend to lack fruits and vegetables in their diet, which are the majority of foods that provide vitamin C. Not to mention that any fruits and vegetables they do consume can be malabsorbed. Vitamin C quickly decreases with stress and infections and becuase people with IBD experience both of these, they can go through the small amount of vitamin C they may be getting too quickly. Antioxidants, such as vitamin C, appear to play a special role in protecting the intestinal cells from inflammation, so it is important to ensure you are getting what your body needs.

Body basics

This vitamin helps to boost the immune system, produce collagen to hold bones and muscles together, keeps blood vessels healthy, helps to absorb iron, aids in wound healing, produces healthy gums, and also helps to protect from infections. The DRI for vitamin C for adult females is 75 mg, and for adult males it is 90 mg. Vitamin C is non-toxic but very high intakes from supplements can cause diarrhea, so you need to be extra careful with supplemental intake of this vitamin. The Upper Tolerable limit to be aware of is 2,000 mg.

Best food sources

The richest sources of vitamin C are fruits and vegetables. Some fruits and vegetables with the highest amounts of vitamin C include citrus fruits, strawberries, kiwi, pineapple, red peppers, potatoes, broccoli, green leafy vegetables, and tomatoes.

| Tip | Antioxidants are substances that help to protect the cells in our body from the effects of free radicals. Free radicals are molecules that are produced when your body digests food, or they can come from environmental exposures such as tobacco smoke, pollution, and radiation. Free radicals damage our body's cells and may play a role in heart disease, cancer, and other illnesses. Antioxidants include beta-carotene, vitamin C, vitamin A, Vitamin E, selenium, lutein, and lycopene. Antioxidants can be found in an abundance of foods, from fruits and veggies to nuts, grains, and even some meats, poultry, and fish. |

Folic acid/folate

Folic acid is in the B family of vitamins. Though many vitamins can pose problems, in the case of deficiencies for people with IBD there are a few that are more problematic than others such as folic acid. *Folic acid* is the synthetic form of this vitamin found in fortified foods and supplements; *folate* is the natural form of this vitamin found naturally in foods. Our body cannot make folate as it can some other nutrients so we must get it from the foods we eat and from supplements.

Many people with IBD have low levels of folate in their blood. This can be due to medications they may be taking to treat their IBD, especially sulfasalzine or methotrexate, because they tend to interfere with the metabolism of folate and folic acid. In addition, people who have Crohn's disease that affects their small intestines are at risk for malabsorption of this vitamin. Those with IBD that have poor appetites and are not eating well can be at risk for a folate deficiency if not being properly supplemented. If you are taking a folic acid supplement for a long period of time, your doctor should also be monitoring your B12 levels, as taking folic acid can mask a B12 deficiency or anemia.

Body basics

Folate is a vitamin that is essential for cell division, red blood cell production and prevention of anemia, production of DNA (our genetic make-up), helping protect against heart disease, and reducing the risk for neural tube birth defects in newborns. Folate is necessary for maintaining proper levels of an amino acid called homocysteine in the body, which is needed for protein synthesis. Without enough folate, homocysteine will build up and these higher levels are associated with cardiovascular or heart disease. Folate deficiencies can cause anemia, low energy levels, lack of appetite, pale looking skin, sore tongue, irritability, and diarrhea.

The DRI for folate is 400 mcg for adults, both male and female. To prevent a folate deficiency, those who are at risk may need extra folic acid. Check with your doctor to determine how much folic acid you need daily. The Tolerable Upper Limit to be aware of for folic acid, the supplemental type, is 1,000 mcg.

Best food sources

Even if you are taking a supplement of folic acid to prevent a deficiency it is still imperative to support the body with adequate nutrient intake from foods as much as possible. Good sources of folate include green leafy vegetables, avocado, legumes, most beans, lentils, whole grains, oranges, fortified breakfast cereals and other fortified foods, and wheat germ.

> **Tip**
>
> If you have IBD and are planning on becoming pregnant you should discuss the need for additional folic acid with your doctor. To prevent the risk for neural tube defects, such as spina bifida, in unborn children, it is essential to resolve any deficiencies and maintain adequate levels of folic acid before you decide to become pregnant.

Vitamin B12

Vitamin B12, known as cobalamin, is also part of the B family of vitamins. Vitamin B12 is absorbed in the small intestines. Those with Crohn's disease, especially those with inflammation in the ileum or the lower part of the small intestines, or those who have had small intestine resections involving the ileum, are at greater risk for B12 deficiencies. This is because the ileum is the area of the small intestines that absorbs all of the vitamin B12 to be used by the body. For these people, vitamin B12 may have a hard time being absorbed not just from food but also even from supplements taken by mouth. People in this situation usually need to get B12 injections on a regular basis to avoid the development of deficiencies. In addition, improper food intake, diarrhea, loss of cells that secrete intrinsic factor (necessary for B12 absorption), and certain medications can lead to a deficiency. For others who don't have issues in that area of the small intestines, consuming a diet with adequate protein and fortified foods will usually provide enough of this B vitamin to sustain health.

Body basics

Vitamin B12 is essential to many bodily functions, including metabolism, DNA synthesis, maintenance of the central nervous system, neurological function, and production of red blood cells. B12, like the other B vitamins, is a water-soluble vitamin and, therefore, any excess that is not used by the body is excreted in the urine. A deficiency of B12 has many of the same symptoms as a folate deficiency, including anemia, but also includes neurological symptoms such as tingling and numbness in the hands or feet, loss of balance, mental changes, and in severe cases even dementia. Other deficiency symptoms include diarrhea, fatigue, loss of appetite, pale skin, and problems concentrating.

The DRI for vitamin B12 is 2.4 mcg for adults, both male and female. Because there is such low potential for toxicity from excess vitamin B12, an Upper Tolerable Limit has not yet been established.

Tip People who have pernicious anemia lack the intrinsic factor necessary for vitamin B12 to be absorbed in the body so these people cannot properly absorb the vitamin. This type of anemia is usually treated with vitamin B12 shots.

Best food sources

Vitamin B12 can naturally be found in animal products such as fish and seafood, meat, poultry, eggs, milk, and milk products. You generally won't find B12 in plant foods such as fruits and vegetables, but you will find it in fortified breakfast cereals and other fortified foods. Fortified foods vary greatly in their content of nutrients, so it is important to read food labels to determine which added nutrients they may contain.

Mighty minerals

Minerals, like vitamins, are a mighty bunch of essential nutrients that are needed to regulate many bodily processes. Unlike vitamins, minerals are inorganic and tend to be much tougher in nature. They cannot be destroyed by heat or food handling methods the way vitamins can. Minerals are first absorbed into the intestines. Some minerals pass directly into the bloodstream and then into body cells, with excess being passed through the urine. Other minerals are carried by being attached to proteins and becoming a part of the body's structure. These types are stored, so excess amounts over long periods of time can be harmful. Minerals come in two different categories: major and trace. The difference between the two is that major minerals are needed by the body in greater amounts than trace minerals are. Both types are essential for optimal health and proper functioning of the body.

Major Minerals	Trace Minerals
Calcium	Iron
Phosphorus	Manganese
Magnesium	Copper
Sodium	Iodine
Potassium	Zinc
Chloride	Cobalt
Sulfur	Fluoride
	Selenium
	Chromium
	Molybdenum

A few other minerals, including boron, nickel, arsenic, silicon, and vanadium, have not yet been deemed necessary for health by nutrition experts.

When it comes to IBD there are a few minerals that can pose deficiency problems. Iron deficiency can be fairly common in people with Crohn's disease or ulcerative colitis. Other minerals deficiencies can include calcium, magnesium, potassium, and zinc.

Iron

Iron may be considered a trace mineral, but it is a powerhouse just the same. Iron is absorbed in the top part of the small intestines called the duodenum. Both people with Crohn's disease and those with ulcerative colitis are prone to iron deficiency for various reasons. Because IBD is associated with both bleeding and malabsorption, it is essential to regulate and measure blood iron levels regularly for these people.

Body basics

Iron has many important functions in the body. A good part of this trace mineral can be found in a protein in red blood cells known as *hemoglobin* that carries about 70 percent of the iron found in the body. It serves as a delivery service, transporting oxygen from your lungs to every part of the body that needs it, such as tissues and organs. Iron is also necessary for brain development and a healthy immune system. Our body depends on iron reserves to produce the normal amounts of blood we need. As the stores of iron become low it can lead to a condition known as iron-deficiency anemia, which can result in fatigue, weakness, irritability, headaches, decreased immune function, and the feeling of being cold. Anemia is a common complication of IBD, with iron deficiency being the predominant cause. Iron deficiency can be caused by low dietary intake of iron, chronic intestinal bleeding, blood loss in the stool, or inadequate absorption, especially in those who have Crohn's disease, and inflammation in the top part of the small intestines.

The DRI for iron is 8 mg for adult males, 18 mg for women 19 to 50 years of age, and 8 mg for women 51 years and older, though the need may be much great for those with IBD. However, too much iron can cause considerable potential for toxicity because very little iron is excreted from the body. The Upper Tolerable Limit for the average person is 45 mg for adults. People on iron supplements should be closely supervised by their doctor.

If your doctor suspects you may be at risk for iron deficiency you may be prescribed a daily iron supplement. Take this as prescribed, which will usually be in two or three equally spaced doses for best absorption and minimizing side effects. Your doctor will evaluate you individually for the amount you need to avoid anemia as well as toxicity, and will monitor your blood levels regularly. Keep in mind that therapeutic doses of iron supplements can cause gastrointestinal side effects such as nausea, cramping, constipation, black stools, and diarrhea, so speak with your doctor if you experience anything unusual. Many times starting with a smaller dose and working your way up can help to minimize these side effects. In addition, taking your supplement with food can help. In rare situations, iron may need to be administered through injection or IV.

Best food sources

Iron can be found in a variety of food sources from animal to plant sources. There are two forms of dietary iron: heme and nonheme. Heme iron is the most absorbable form of iron found in foods and is only available in animal sources such as red meats, fish, seafood, and poultry. Nonheme iron is not quite as absorbable and is found in plant foods such as lentils and beans. This is usually the form of iron added to iron-enriched and iron-fortified foods. Consuming nonheme iron sources along with foods high in vitamin C can give them a boost of absorbability.

Calcium

Calcium is the most abundant mineral in our bodies, with almost 99 percent being stored in the tissues of the bones and in the teeth. Calcium is found in some foods, is added to others, can be found as a dietary supplement, and can even be found in some medicines such as antacids. For various reasons people with IBD can be prone to a deficiency of this all-too-important mineral.

Body basics

Calcium gives our bones and teeth strength, helps slow the rate of bone loss as we age, and helps muscles contract and the heart beat. Calcium regulates blood pressure, regulates nerve transmission, and helps blood clot. The body uses the bones to store calcium and takes if from there to regulate concentrations of calcium in the blood.

A calcium deficiency won't show any obvious symptoms in the short term the way iron might. Calcium in the blood is tightly regulated and taken from bone tissue if needed. If this is done too often, over the long term, osteopenia or softening of the bones can occur, and if left untreated can lead to osteoporosis. This increases the risk of bone fractures. People with IBD may be deficient in calcium intake due to poor dietary intake from lack of appetite, not absorbing enough calcium from foods, being lactose intolerant (avoiding all dairy products), or certain medications. Some people can have symptoms from a calcium deficiency (if it is severe enough) primarily from medical problems or treatments that could result in numbness and tingling in the fingers, muscle cramps, lethargy, poor appetite, and abnormal heart rhythms.

The DRI for calcium for adult males is 1,000 mg from 19 to 70 years of age and 1,200 mg at 71 years and older. Adult females are recommended 1,000 mg from 19 to 50 years and 1,200 mg at 51 years and older. High calcium intake can cause kidney problems, constipation, and inadequate zinc and iron absorption. The Upper Tolerable Limit to be aware of is between 2,000 and 2,500 mg. Speak with your doctor about the dosage of this supplement that is right for you, as calcium supplements have the potential to interact with some medications.

> **Tip** There are two main forms of calcium supplements: carbonate and citrate. Both are absorbed well but individuals with reduced levels of stomach acid can absorb the citrate form more easily. The carbonate form is more efficiently absorbed when taken with food whereas the citrate form can be taken with or without food to be equally absorbed. The amount of elemental calcium in a supplement is the part that is actually absorbed. Calcium carbonate is 40 percent calcium; citrate is 21 percent calcium. Check labels on your supplements to find out how much calcium you are truly getting. Absorption is best in doses of less than 500 mg at a time. Some people may experience GI side effects from calcium supplements though carbonate tends to cause more of these side effects then citrate.

Best food sources

Most popularly when we think about calcium we automatically think about milk and other dairy products such as yogurt and cheese, which are excellent sources of calcium. Calcium can also be found in canned sardines and salmon with edible bones, broccoli, legumes, almonds, dried figs, dark green leafy vegetables, calcium-fortified tofu, and other calcium-fortified foods such as orange juice, cereal, and soy milk.

Magnesium

Magnesium is essential to good health, with approximately 50 percent of it found in our bones. The other half is found mostly inside cells, tissues, and organs. Magnesium is also one of the electrolytes, which are nutrients that play a vital role in maintaining balance within the body. Electrolytes help to regulate heart and neurological function, fluid balance, oxygen delivery, acid-base balance, and much more. It is the balance of these electrolytes that is essential for normal function. When deficiencies of electrolytes occur, it causes an imbalance in the body. Besides magnesium, sodium, potassium, and chloride are also classified as electrolytes.

Body basics

Magnesium helps maintain normal muscle and nerve function, helps keep the heart's rhythm steady, supports a healthy immune system, and keeps bones strong. Magnesium also plays a part in regulating blood sugar levels and promoting normal blood pressure, and is involved in energy metabolism. For those with Crohn's disease and/or chronic diarrhea (causes loss of electrolytes), it can be hard to get all of the magnesium your body needs. A deficiency of this mineral is not uncommon in IBD but can be hard to detect. If you are dealing with extreme diarrhea, though, then you are at greater risk. Deficiency symptoms can include loss of appetite, nausea, vomiting, fatigue, and weakness. Symptoms can worsen if the deficiency worsens with numbness, tingling, muscle contractions and cramps, mental changes, abnormal heart rhythms, and coronary spasms.

The Adequate Intake (AI) for magnesium for males 19 to 30 years is 400 mg and for males 31 years and older is 420 mg. The AI for females 19 to 30 years is 310 mg and for females 31 years and older is 320 mg. Too much magnesium only comes from supplementation and can also cause problems such as diarrhea, abdominal cramping, nausea, loss of appetite, muscle weakness, difficulty breathing, very low blood pressure, and irregular heartbeat. The last thing you need if you are already having problems with diarrhea is more, so the best way to try to supplement is with food and a moderate multivitamin/mineral supplement unless otherwise prescribed by your doctor. The Upper Tolerable Limit to be aware of is 350 mg for adults.

Best food sources

Diets high in vegetables (especially green vegetables), fruits, legumes, nuts, seeds, and whole grains tend to be adequate in magnesium. Meat and dairy products are poor sources of this mineral.

Potassium and zinc

Here's a quick mention about potassium and zinc, both of which can cause deficiency problems. Potassium is an important mineral and is involved in the proper functioning of all cells, tissues, and organs in the body. Potassium is also an electrolyte and is one of the more serious electrolyte disturbances when there is an abnormality in its levels. Chronic diarrhea and/or vomiting can lead to electrolyte imbalances along with dehydration. Potassium is crucial to heart function and muscle contraction (including digestive muscles). For those with IBD, deficiencies may develop from diarrhea, vomiting, malnutrition, or inadequate absorption, and/or as a result of some medications such as prednisone. Too little potassium is known as hypokalemia, and too much potassium in the blood is known as hyperkalemia. Keeping the right balance depends on the amount of other electrolytes in the body, including sodium, chloride, and magnesium. The AI for potassium is 4.7 grams for adults. No Upper Tolerable Limit has been established. Good dietary sources of potassium include bananas, citrus fruits and juices, avocados, cantaloupes, tomatoes, potatoes, salmon, chicken, and other meats. Because there are potential side effects and interactions with medications, only take potassium supplements under the direct supervision of your doctor.

Zinc is an essential mineral that is involved in cellular metabolism, is required for the activity of many enzymes, and plays a role in immune function, protein synthesis, wound healing, DNA synthesis, and cell division. In addition, zinc is essential for normal growth and development during pregnancy. The body doesn't store zinc, so constant supply is needed. People with IBD can experience a deficiency of zinc mainly from insufficient intake, poor absorption, and diarrhea. Some of the most common deficiency symptoms of zinc include loss of appetite, impaired immune function, and growth retardation. If the deficiency is severe enough one might also experience hair loss, diarrhea, impotence, delayed sexual maturation, and eye and skin lesions, as well as weight loss, impaired wound healing, taste abnormalities, and mental lethargy. Many of these symptoms, as with all of the vitamin and mineral deficiencies we have discussed, are most of the time non-specific and can be associated with other health conditions, including IBD. Therefore it is important to undergo a medical examination and laboratory blood work before assumption of a deficiency is made. The DRI for zinc for adult females is 8 mg, and for adult males that increases to 11 mg daily. You can get too much zinc, so be aware that the Upper Tolerable Limit is 40 mg for both adult males and adult females. A wide variety of foods supply zinc, including oysters (which contains more zinc then any other food), red meat, poultry, beans, nuts, some seafood, whole grains, fortified breakfast cereals, and dairy products.

> **Tip** The Upper Tolerable Limits set by the National Academy of Sciences, Institute of Medicine and Food and Nutrition Board do not necessarily apply to individuals receiving supplemental therapy for medical treatment but such individuals should be under close supervision by their doctors to monitor for possible adverse health effects.

When Supplements Are Necessary

Because the majority of the people with IBD have problems absorbing enough nutrients from foods and with eating enough food, it is a good bet that you will need nutritional supplementation. Depending on the extent and location of your disease along with your risk for nutrient deficiencies, your doctor may prescribe nutritional supplements. Because your nutritional needs may vary depending on whether you are experiencing a flare-up or whether you are in remission, it is best to consult with your doctor and a dietitian before taking supplements or altering your diet on your own.

Absorbability is a critical factor when it comes to taking vitamin/mineral supplements for people with IBD. Hard tablets may not break down as easily, so they may not be as effective as liquid supplements or liquid or powder-filled capsules, which are both much more quickly metabolized and better absorbed. It is important that your supplement is a high-quality product to ensure you are getting what you need. Again, speak with your doctor about a supplement that will work best for you.

In addition to nutritional supplements, a fiber supplement may be needed, depending on your specific condition, where you are in the progression of your disease (active/remission), and how severe your disease is. During an acute flare-up fiber is usually something to back off of a bit, but at other times it may be beneficial. In some people fiber supplements such as psyllium powder can help to stop mild diarrhea. Not all fiber supplements are created equal. They are mainly made of psyllium, methylcellulose, or polycarbophil. Each type of supplement can vary in its properties, uses, and side effects. Talk to your doctor about which might be best for your body and situation. When taking fiber supplements, always start at a low dose, working your way up, and drink plenty of water.

Chapter 7

Alternative Treatments to Discover

Because IBD is a chronic condition, people who are afflicted need to find ongoing treatments to continuously manage their illness throughout their life. For some people, conventional medical treatments such as medications and surgery may not offer them as much relief as they would like. Complementary and alternative medicine (CAM) approaches can offer people additional choices to feeling better and living a more normal life. Most experts recommend using CAM approaches in addition to traditional approaches rather than as replacements. It is ultimately up to you and your doctor whether CAM approaches should be part of your treatment plan for IBD. The science behind these types of therapies for IBD varies greatly, with some having quality research studies to support their effectiveness and others having research that is only based on a small number of people without controlled research trials. Most CAM therapies are safe to use with conventional medical treatment except for possible herbal supplements because some can interact with medications as well as come with side effects. It is very important to always speak with your doctor before adding any type of complementary or alternative treatment method to your current medical treatment plan.

Discovering Omega-3 Fats

Before you can understand how omega-3 fats may help IBD you need to know what they are. An omega-3 fatty acid is a type of polyunsaturated fat that is not made in the body but is found in foods. Foods highest in omega-3 fats include fattier fish such as salmon, herring, halibut, lake trout, mackerel, albacore tuna, and sardines. In fish, omega-3 fats are found in the forms of EPA (eicosapentaeonic) and DHA (docoshexaeonic), which provide the greatest health benefits. They can also be found in a less-potent form called ALA (alpha linolenic acid), which is a precursor for EPA and DHA in some plant sources including walnuts, ground flaxseed, canola oil, numerous nut oils, pumpkin seeds, and soybeans. You can also boost your intake of omega-3 fatty acids by taking fish oil supplements. However, too much in the form of supplements can have health implications for some people, so speak with your doctor first.

> **Tip**
>
> You can find new foods on the market today that are fortified with omega-3 fatty acids such as eggs, yogurt, peanut butter, margarine, bread, and pasta. Be aware that these fortified foods usually contain very little omega-3 fat and you would need to eat a lot of the food to get close to what is recommended. Additional omega-3 fatty acids found in these foods aren't harmful but don't substitute these "functional foods" for ones that naturally contain omega-3 fatty acids.

Omega-3 fats play a crucial role in brain function as well as normal growth and development of the body. Research has also shown these fats to help reduce inflammation, as well as the risk for heart disease, certain cancers, and arthritis. They can help to lower total cholesterol, increase good cholesterol, lower triglycerides, lower blood pressure, improve some skin disorders, help alleviate symptoms of depression as well as other psychological disorders, and the list goes on.

Omega-3 fats are being studied as a complementary treatment for IBD possibly due to their anti-inflammatory affects. Some research has suggested that fish oil may be effective in reducing existing inflammation but not necessarily in preventing inflammation. In addition, numerous studies have found that omega-3 fats might also help to reduce the risk of relapse, repair tissue damage, and improve IBD symptoms. At this point, results have been mixed, but it is known that these fats in general are a healthy addition to any diet. The American Heart Association (AHA) recommends that the general public eat fish (particularly fatty fish) at least two times (two 3.5-ounce servings) per week.

The bottom line is that more research needs to be done to determine the extent of anti-inflammatory properties and other effects on IBD, but so far they look quite promising. Consider adding fattier fish to your diet and speak with your doctor about whether a fish oil supplement will fit into your treatment plan. The optimal amount of omega-3 fat in the diet has not been defined for IBD, so your doctor will need to make that recommendation.

Tip

When choosing a fish oil supplement, take a good look at the label on the bottle. Just because a supplement lists 1 gram or 1,000 mg of fish oil doesn't mean it is all coming from omega-3 fatty acids. The amount of EPA and DHA is the most important component because these are the true indicators of the amount of healthy omega-3 fatty acids in the supplement. For example, if the label states the 1,000 mg fish oil supplement contains 250 mg of EPA and 250 mg of DHA then it has a total of 500 mg of omega-3 fatty acids, not 1,000 mg. The key is not to look for total oil content in the capsule but instead the amount of EPA and DHA per serving.

If you want to add fish and seafood to your diet for its health benefits but the mercury content is a concern, then listen up. You most definitely do not need to avoid fish due to mercury, but if you are a woman who may become pregnant, a pregnant woman, or a nursing mom, or you have young children, you should know which fish to choose and how much. The advisory by the U.S. FDA (Food and Drug Administration) and the U.S. EPA (Environmental Protection Agency) states for this population:

- Do not eat shark, swordfish, king mackerel, or tilefish because they contain higher levels of mercury.

- Eat up to 12 ounces (two average meals) a week of a variety of fish and shellfish that are lower in mercury. Five of the most commonly eaten fish, low in mercury, are shrimp, canned light tuna, salmon, pollock, and catfish. Albacore (white) tuna has more mercury then canned light tuna; you may eat up to 6 ounces of albacore tuna per week.

- Check local advisories about the safety of fish if caught by family and friends in your local lakes, rivers, and coastal areas. If you cannot find advice, eat up to 6 ounces per week of fish you catch from local waters, and do not consume any other fish that week.

These same recommendations hold true for young children, but they are to be served smaller portions.

Even with these recommendations in mind, the recommendation by the AHA for omega-3 fatty acids is to eat two servings of fish per week and at 3 to 4 ounces per serving, which is well below the FDA and EPA's safe limit of 12 ounces per week. Eating a variety of fish and following the recommendations will ensure that you can still enjoy fish, feel safe, and enjoy all its healthy benefits. For more information on this advisory and about mercury and contaminant content of fish go to: *www.epa.gov/fishadvisories/advice*.

Find Out About Flaxseed Oil

Flaxseed oil comes from the seeds of the flax plant and contains both omega-3 and omega-6 fats. Flaxseed contains the ALA form of omega-3 fats that is converted into EPA and DHA, which are the forms found in fish oil. The body isn't quite as efficient at converting ALA into EPA and DHA, so it isn't quite as potent as the omega-3 fats found in fish and fish oil. Preliminary studies have found that the ALA such as that found in flaxseed may help to reduce bowel inflammation, but results are mixed on its effectiveness. In addition, recent studies have shown positive benefits that flaxseed oil may help to heal the inner lining of an inflamed intestines. Moderate intake of flaxseed oil and ground flaxseed may offer some benefit. Talk to your doctor before adding flaxseed or flaxseed oil to your diet, because it can slow down the absorption of some oral medications and other nutrients if taken at the same time.

Benefits of Probiotics

A complementary aid in the treatment of IBD called "probiotics" is increasing in popularity and proving to possibly be beneficial. Probiotic therapy may help to ease symptoms of IBD and promote the body's own self-healing process. Probiotics are non-harmful, living, "good" or "friendly" bacteria that can naturally be found in your intestines and can aid in digestion. It is assumed that it is "bad" bacteria in the gut that eventually leads to triggering inflammatory cells that trigger IBD. Experts believe that adding "good" bacteria to the gut can help minimize the effect of harmful or "bad" bacteria by keeping the flora in the gut in better balance. This basically means that probiotics can help to reduce the number of bad bacteria that adhere to the intestinal wall, which in turn helps to reduce inflammation. It seems that when the balance between "good" and "bad" bacteria is thrown off, it can cause all types of GI disturbances. New studies are looking into the role probiotics play as a therapeutic option for IBD. Studies are testing the use of probiotics in helping to reduce symptoms and achieve remission in IBD flare-ups. At this point, most studies are still inconclusive about whether these substances can help, but research continues.

Probiotics can be found in capsule form or in a drink or food. In fact, the easiest food to find them in is yogurt where active or live bacterial cultures have been added. Unfortunately with these products there is no standardization so you don't always know how much or what kind you are getting. At the least, look for yogurts that state "contain" live active cultures on the container as opposed to those that state "made with" live active cultures. The most widely used probiotics include *bifidobacterium* and *lactobacillus*.

Tip

Extensive studies on products such as *VSL#3*, *Culturally,* and *OMX Probiotic 12+* have shown a positive effect on reducing IBD. Therapeutic doses may be needed and different strains of probiotics have different effects so if you are interested in trying probiotics speak with your doctor to find out what might work for you.

Advantages of Prebiotics

New research is also currently looking into the benefits of prebiotic supplements on IBD. Prebiotics are non-digestible carbohydrates that are fermented by bacteria in the colon. This fermentation provides the energy for the growth of "good" bacteria, which again can help balance the "good" and "bad" bacteria in the gut. Your body doesn't digest prebiotics so they remain in your digestive tract, and there they stimulate the growth of beneficial bacteria and keep it healthy. Examples of prebiotics include fructooligosaccharides (FOS), inulin, lactulose, and galactooligosaccharides. Prebiotics can be found in foods such as onions, garlic, bananas, asparagus, artichokes, leeks, and wheat. Some companies are now adding prebiotics to food supplements. FOS may be added to foods or can be taken as a supplement. If you are following a FODMAP approach, you need to be extra careful with both probiotics and prebiotics.

> **Tip** Speak to your doctor before taking a prebiotic and limit your intake, as prebiotics can cause gas and cramping. In addition, if you need to take an antibiotic to fight an infection you may need to adjust your intake of prebiotics and probiotics, because these medications tend to kill off "good" bacteria, allowing "bad" bacteria to take over the gut flora, which can lead to more problems for people with IBD.

Potential Herbal Remedies

A popular complementary therapy among people with IBD is herbal remedies. However, it is important to know that they should only complement and never replace your conventional medical treatment. Although there are many herbal remedies out there that tout their benefits for IBD, we will just talk about a few of the most popular ones.

Boswellia

Boswellia is an herb that comes from the resin of the bark of the *Boswellian serrata* tree, which is native to India. This herb is commonly used to lessen the symptoms of IBD. In addition, the anti-inflammatory properties of boswellia extracts seem to be effective in possibly helping to control the inflammation involved with IBD as well as other inflammatory conditions. Boswellia rarely causes side effects, but if it does you can end up with diarrhea, nausea, and/or a skin rash. Boswellia can be found in pill form and the label should state that it is standardized to contain at least 60 percent boswellic acids. It should not be taken long term, only for 8 to 12 weeks, and should only be taken under your doctor's supervision.

Bromelain

Bromelain is an enzyme that is derived from the juice and stems of pineapple. This herb is believed to help with the digestion of protein as well as help reduce inflammation, making it popular for people with IBD and other inflammatory disorders. Studies have found that taking bromelain on a regular basis may decrease the severity of colitis.

> **Tip**
>
> The use of herbs has been around for many years and even though they are thought of as a natural therapy, they do contain active substances that can trigger side effects and interact with other herbs, supplements, and medications. For this reason always speak with your doctor before taking *any* type of herbal remedy, natural or not. Herbs should be taken with care and always under the supervision of your doctor.

Bromelain is usually extracted from pineapple and formulated into a capsule or tablet. When used as an anti-inflammatory, most experts typically suggest taking bromelain between meals on an empty stomach to maximize its absorption. Some of the more common side effects of taking bromelain include diarrhea, nausea, and indigestion. It may also cause vomiting, increased heart rate, drowsiness, and changes in menstruation. Bromelain has been found to cause allergic reactions and asthma symptoms as well. People with allergies including pineapple, rye, wheat, papain, bee venom, grass, and certain pollens should not take bromelain. People with peptic ulcers should also not take bromelain. If you suffer from a digestive disorder, speak with your doctor before taking this herbal supplement. Bromelain can increase bleeding and is not proven safe for pregnant and nursing women, as well as children and people with liver or kidney disease. Bromelain can interfere with some medications as well.

Slippery elm

Slippery elm comes from the bark of the slippery elm tree. It has been used for many, many years to treat diarrhea and other gastrointestinal problems. This herb is believed to possess anti-inflammatory and antioxidant properties. Though there hasn't been enough significant research to support the theory to this point, the research that has been done seems promising. The belief is that slippery elm contains a substance called mucilage, which most plants contain, that is found in higher amounts in this plant. Supposedly when taken orally, mucilage coats the mucous membranes in the GI tract, including the stomach, and helps to soothe inflammation and relieve pain. In addition, studies are being done to help confirm the antioxidant effects of slippery elm on helping to relieve inflammatory bowel conditions.

It is the inner bark of the slippery elm tree that is dried and turned into powder and used for medicinal purposes. This herb comes in tablets, capsules, lozenges, and a fine powder for making teas or extracts. As with all other herbs, precautions should be taken when taking slippery elm. This herb can possibly slow down the digestive process, which can prevent the proper absorption of some medications, supplements, and/or other herbs, so they should not be taken at the same time. At this point slippery elm has not been found to interact with any medications or cause any serious side effects, but research of this is ongoing. As with any medication or herb there is always a chance of allergic reaction. It is not yet confirmed whether this herb is safe for women who are pregnant or breastfeeding. At this point in time slippery elm has not been approved by the FDA to treat any specific medical conditions. Always check with your doctor before taking this or any other herbal supplement.

Aloe vera

Aloe vera is a plant that has been used for many centuries to treat all types of conditions. This herb has an anti-inflammatory effect as well as possibly acting as an antifungal and antibacterial agent. The gel of the plant leaves is used widely for wound healing and pain relief. Although it has not been extensively studied for IBD, some people take it in a liquid juice form to help treat mild to moderate symptoms of ulcerative colitis.

As with other herbs, allergic reactions are possible in some people. The safety of aloe vera has not been established for use in children, pregnant or breastfeeding women, or people with liver and kidney disease. The form known as aloe latex or drug aloe has strong laxative effects and should not be used by people with intestinal disorders such as IBD. This form of aloe can cause problems if you take too much and should not be taken for longer than 10 days. It can also cause potential drug interactions. As always, check with your doctor before considering adding aloe vera to your supplement list.

Alternative Coping Strategies

The complementary treatment options we talked about in the chapter so far are more for the physical part of IBD. It is important though to treat yourself as a whole, and that involves both body and mind. Your mind and body are so closely interrelated that emotional stress can influence the course and severity of your disease. Emotional distress such as stress, anxiety, and tension does not cause IBD but happens most likely as a reaction to the symptoms of the disease itself. In addition, that emotional stress can certainly influence the frequency and severity of flare-ups and its symptoms.

It can take time to adjust to accepting your disease and to living with IBD in your own way. It is vital to give yourself time and to be open to the different options that are out there for you. Although IBD is a serious and chronic condition, it is not considered fatal, and most people with IBD can still live a happy, useful, and productive life. But it is up to you to do the best you can to make that happen. Learning to cope, taking an active role in your care, and maintaining a positive outlook can make a world of difference. It won't happen overnight but, if you give yourself a chance to be proactive, it can happen. There is never a reason to feel alone or helpless unless you let yourself. First and foremost, follow the treatment plan and medications your doctor has planned for you. You can speak with a therapist who is knowledgeable about IBD and/or chronic illnesses, and/or become involved in local support groups full of people that are in your same situation and can offer support and help with coping strategies.

In addition to those coping strategies, looking at alternative ways to decrease your stress, anxiety, and tension is also an option. We talked a bit about exercise, meditation, and yoga earlier in the book, all great ways to decrease stress and help you feel more empowered when it comes to your own health. But there are a few others that you might want to consider and explore. These therapies are no miracle cure of any kind, but they can possibly help, along with medical treatment, to relieve symptoms, reduce the frequency of flare-ups, decrease your emotional stress, as well as empower you to feel you are doing something to help yourself. Only you can decide what is right for you. Check out the Resource Guide.

Attempting acupuncture

Acupuncture is an ancient Chinese technique used to heal pain, stress, and other ailments. It is one of the most studied CAM therapies. Acupuncture is based on the belief that the human body's vital energy flow, or "chi," flows along certain pathways in the body and needs to be in balance for the body to be healthy and function properly. Depending on the ailment, different sizes of thin, sharp needles are gently inserted into specific acupuncture points on the body to stimulate and rebalance the body's energy in those areas. This is meant to release special hormones that trigger the natural healing process to let the body properly do its work. In addition, acupuncture is said to help regulate blood flow and help release endorphins that can in turn help to relieve pain. Traditional acupuncture therapy is believed to treat the body as a whole and to regulate emotional, mental, spiritual, and physical balance. Even though the thought of needles may make you cringe, it is quite painless, with few side effects, if any. Acupuncture itself is safe regardless of a person's health and/or medications, however, many times acupuncture is used in combination with herbal therapies, and those can be contraindicated for certain health issues and medications being taken. In most states, acupuncture is a licensed profession and the therapist must be board certified, so do your homework before you choose one to visit.

Recent studies have found that acupuncture may have some benefits when it comes to gastrointestinal diseases such as IBD. A few studies have found that the overall quality of life for people with IBD improved significantly with regular acupuncture treatments.

Researching Reiki therapy

You may have never heard of it, but Reiki is an ancient form of natural Japanese healing that has actually been around for many centuries. The term *Reiki* actually means "spiritually guided life energy" or more commonly "universal life energy." Treatments are based on the channeling and balancing of positive energy within the body, through a practitioner, to promote overall health and healing. Reiki therapy sends the body into a deep state of relaxation, which is said to unlock the body's own healing powers. This type of therapy is meant to address physical, emotional, mental, and spiritual imbalance

Reiki is full of a variety of benefits including reducing stress and anxiety levels, increasing energy levels, improving the immune system, and reducing muscle pain. There is nothing you have to do during a Reiki treatment except to have an open mind to trying it. During a Reiki session the practitioner uses gentle hand movements to channel positive energy from his or her hands to that of the patient. Hand movements hover just above the patient's body and are often performed without body contact, depending on whether other therapies are being used in conjunction with Reiki. When you receive a Reiki treatment specifically for your condition, the practitioner will focus on balancing the energy in the areas of the body that are of concern. These regions are called chakras. Chakras are energy centers within the body where it is believed that energy enters and leaves the body, and also where healing energies can get stuck or clogged. Reiki energy needs to be able to flow freely through the body. If it can't, then the regions located in the area of the energy block can cease to function properly. A Reiki treatment is probably one of the most relaxing treatments you will ever experience and one worth a try. Be sure to seek a Reiki therapist who is properly trained and qualified by inquiring about schooling, qualifications, and training.

Chapter 8

Delicious and Helpful Recipes

Learning about all of the foods that do and don't trigger IBD flare-ups and symptoms for you is one thing, but learning how to focus on the foods you can have and including them every day can be another. Life can get busy and hectic, and it can be easy to stray from those healthy foods we know are safer. Planning ahead is key. Planning your weekly meals and menus before you grocery shop will make things much easier. Stock your pantry, refrigerator, and freezer with only healthy foods you know you can tolerate so you don't tempt yourself to reach for something that might be trouble. Keep foods on hand for those times when you experience a flare-up and getting out to the store isn't an option.

To help give you a head start, I have included a variety of recipes from other nutritional professionals that can add nutritional value and great flavor to your daily meal plans. Keep in mind that everyone with IBD is different with regard to which foods they can and can't tolerate, so use the recipes as a start and substitute foods as needed. Some of these recipes will be a food fit when you might be in remission, and others might work well during flare-ups. Use your own judgment by knowing which foods work best for you at certain times. Hopefully using some of these recipes will motivate you to take it a step further and experiment with other nutritious recipes from books, friends, family, support groups, and on-line, or even to create your own tasty recipes. Let these recipes be a start to better managing your diet and helping to boost your nutritional intake. Just because you have IBD doesn't mean you have to eat a bland, tasteless diet!

Remember that the goal is to eat as much variety as possible to get as many nutrients in as possible, so don't count out foods unless you know for sure they are trouble for you. Again, if you need help in determining which foods work best for you, seek the help of a registered dietitian.

Soups

 Tomato Basil Cream Soup
Makes 6 1-cup servings

1 Tbsp. olive oil
3/4 cup chopped onions
2 garlic cloves, minced
15-oz. can diced tomatoes, no-salt-added
15-oz. can stewed tomatoes
1 1/2 cups low-sodium chicken broth
12 oz. silken tofu
1 Tbs. fresh chopped basil
1/4 tsp. black pepper, to taste

Heat the oil in a large Dutch oven and sauté the onions and garlic until tender, about 3 minutes. Add the rest of the ingredients and bring to a boil. Blend in blender or food processor until smooth. Sprinkle with fresh chopped basil and fresh lime juice just before serving. This would make a nice chilled soup in the summertime.

Nutrition note: This soup is easy on the GI system and an excellent source of vitamin A and vitamin C, as well as a good source of protein.

Nutritional information per serving:

Calories: 114
Total fat: 4 g
Saturated fat: 0.5 g
Carbohydrate: 13 g
Protein: 7.5 g
Cholesterol: 0 mg
Sodium: 322 mg
Dietary fiber: 3 g
Sugars: 8 g

Source: Food and Health Communications
foodandhealth.com

Quick & Creamy Beet Soup
Makes 4 ¾-cup servings

15-oz. can diced beets and juice
1 cup evaporated skim milk
2 Tbsp. apple juice concentrate
1 tsp. balsamic vinegar
½ tsp. dried dill weed

Place the diced beets and their liquid into a blender; add the remaining ingredients. Puree until completely smooth, about 1 minute. Transfer to a medium saucepan and heat gently until steamy. Optional garnish: a dollop of non-fat sour cream.

Nutrition note: Another soup easy on the GI system, and it is a good source of calcium and protein. Beets are an excellent source of folate and a very good source of antioxidants, potassium, vitamin C, iron, magnesium, and phosphorus.

Nutritional information per serving:

Calories: 100
Total fat: 0 g
Saturated fat: 0 g
Carbohydrate: 18 g
Protein: 6 g
Cholesterol: 0 mg
Sodium: 350 mg
Dietary fiber: 1 g
Sugars: 7.3 g

Source: Food and Health Communications
foodandhealth.com

 ## Mushroom-Barley Soup
Makes 6 1-cup servings

1/2 tsp. oil
1 medium onion, diced
2 cups fresh mushrooms, sliced
1/4 cup pearled barley
4 cups water
4 cups chicken or vegetable broth
black pepper to taste
pinch thyme
1 bay leaf

Heat a large soup pan over medium-high heat. Add the oil and sauté the onions and mushrooms until golden, about 3 minutes. Add the rest of the ingredients and bring to a boil. Reduce the heat to low and simmer until the barley is tender, about 90 minutes

Nutrition Note: The perfect soup when you are not feeling your best. It is low in fiber and packs in some protein and healing antioxidants.

Nutritional information per serving:

Calories: 81
Total fat: 2.1 g
Saturated fat: 0.1 g
Carbohydrate: 9.7 g
Protein: 6.8 g
Cholesterol: 16 mg
Sodium: 174 mg
Dietary fiber: 2 g
Sugars: 1.3 g

Source: Food and Health Communications
foodandhealth.com

Entrées

 ## Chicken Rice Casserole
Makes 4 1-cup servings

2 cups cooked white chicken meat, skinless and cut into cubes
1 cup white rice
2 cups low-sodium chicken broth
1 cup frozen mixed vegetables
1 tsp. Italian seasoning

Place all ingredients in 2-quart microwaveable container. Cover and cook on medium power until rice is done, about 20 to 25 minutes. Stir occasionally. Serve hot.

Nutrition note: This comfort food is an excellent source of vitamin A and a good source of iron and calories. It is high in carbs yet low in fiber when you need something a bit more gentle.

Nutritional information per serving:

Calories: 341
Total fat: 3.5 g

Saturated fat: 0.5 g
Carbohydrate: 42.6 g
Protein: 6.8 g
Cholesterol: 78 mg
Sodium: 217 mg
Dietary fiber: 2.2 g
Sugars: 0.2 g

Source: Food and Health Communications
foodandhealth.com

Savory Roast Turkey Breast
Makes 14 3-ounce servings

1 turkey breast (5 to 5-1/2 lb.)
1 medium white onion
2 stalks celery, cut in half
vegetable cooking spray
1 1/2 Tbsp. lemon-pepper seasoning
1 1/2 tsp. onion powder
1 1/2 tsp. garlic powder
1 1/2 tsp. poultry seasoning
1/2 tsp. paprika
1 browning bag

Remove and discard the skin from the turkey breast. Rinse the breast and pat it dry. Place the onion and celery into the breast cavity. Spray it all over with cooking spray. Combine the lemon-pepper seasoning, onion powder, garlic powder, poultry seasoning, and paprika. Sprinkle this mixture over the breast. Place it in a browning bag that has been prepared according to the package directions. Place the bag in a shallow baking pan and bake at 325 degrees for one hour. Cut a slit in the top of the bag and bake until a meat thermometer registers 170 degrees, about one hour. Transfer the breast to a serving platter and let it stand for 15 minutes before carving it into thin slices. Use the pan drippings to make low-fat gravy.

Nutrition note: This easy entrée is an excellent source of lean protein.

Nutritional information per serving:

Calories: 114
Total fat: 0.5 g
Saturated fat: 0 g
Carbohydrate: 0 g
Protein: 25 g
Cholesterol: 70 mg
Sodium: 44 mg
Dietary fiber: 0 g
Sugars: 0.3 g

Source: Food and Health Communications
foodandhealth.com

Smoothies and Shakes

 Creamy Banana Shake
Makes 2 ¾-cup servings

1 banana, peeled
1 cup half and half or skim milk
pinch cinnamon
1 Tbsp. light whipped cream

Place banana, half and half (or milk), and cinnamon in blender. Puree on high speed until smooth. You can sweeten with Splenda, NutraSweet, or honey if desired. Pour into a tall glass and top with whipped cream. Enjoy!

Nutrition note: This easy to make shake is perfect when you are not up to eating solid foods. It is a good source of calcium as well as vitamins A and C. It packs in some calories and carbs, too.

Nutritional information per serving:

Calories: 169
Total fat: 1.5 g
Saturated fat: 1g
Carbohydrate: 20 g
Protein: 2 g
Cholesterol: 24 mg
Sodium: 5 mg
Dietary fiber: 1.5 g
Sugars: 12.3 g

Source: Food and Health Communications
Http://foodandhealth.com

 Rise and Shine! Smoothie
Makes 2   1¼-cup servings

1 cup orange juice
1 cup skim or fortified soy milk
3 Tbsp. wheat germ
1 cup fresh or frozen fruit (strawberries, blueberries, bananas, peaches, etc.)
pinch cinnamon

Place all ingredients in a blender and puree on high speed until smooth. Serve immediately or refrigerate for later use, up to eight hours. If you are making this the night before, I recommend you store it in the blender jar and blend it again quickly before serving.

Nutrition note: A quick, delicious, and nutritious smoothie. It is an excellent source of vitamins A and C as well as a good source of calcium.

Nutritional information per serving:

Calories: 160
Total fat: 1.8 g
Saturated fat: 0 g

Carbohydrate: 20 g
Protein: 4.3 g
Cholesterol: 2 mg
Sodium: 30 mg
Dietary fiber: 1.9 g
Sugars: 22.1 g

Source: Food and Health Communications
foodandhealth.com

 # *Banana Smoothie*
Makes 2 servings

1 cup skim milk
1 banana
1/4 tsp. ground cinnamon
1/8 tsp. ground nutmeg
1 Tbsp. fat-free whipped cream

Place milk, banana, and spices in a blender and blend on high speed until smooth. Top with whipped cream and enjoy!

Nutrition note: Gentle on your system, this quick and easy smoothie is a great source of calcium and potassium, as well as a good source of vitamins A and C.

Nutritional information per serving:

Calories: 94
Total fat: 0 g
Saturated fat: 0 g
Carbohydrate: 19 g
Protein: 5 g
Cholesterol: 3 mg
Sodium: 52 mg
Dietary fiber: 1.5 g
Sugars: 13 g

Source: Food and Health Communications
foodandhealth.com

Breakfast Entrées

 ## *Garden Omelet*
Makes 2 1-cup servings

butter-flavored cooking spray
1/2 cup sliced mushrooms
1/2 cup chopped fresh tomato
1/4 cup chopped onion
6 egg whites
1 tsp. Dijon mustard
1 tsp. tarragon
1/4 tsp. garlic powder
1/8 tsp. white pepper
1 Tbsp. reduced-fat grated Parmesan cheese

Spray a large nonstick skillet with butter-flavored spray and heat over medium-high heat. Brown mushrooms, tomato, and onion in the butter spray.

In a large bowl, beat the rest of the ingredients until foamy. Pour over the browned vegetables and cook over medium heat until puffy and light brown on the bottom, about 5 minutes. Fold the omelet in half and place a lid over the skillet for 5 minutes until the omelet is done. Divide in half and enjoy!

Nutrition note: This quick and healthy omelet is great for any meal if you are looking for something light. It is an excellent source of vitamin C and a good source of vitamin A and protein.

Nutritional information per serving:

Calories: 91
Total fat: 1.5 g
Saturated fat: 0.5 g
Carbohydrate: 6.5 g

Protein: 13 g
Cholesterol: 2 mg
Sodium: 232 mg
Dietary fiber: 1.3 g
Sugars: 2.7 g

Source: Food and Health Communications
foodandhealth.com

 # Cinnamon Apple Millet
Makes about 4 large servings

1 container hemp milk (4 cups)
1 cup dried millet
1 large apple, diced (if FODMAPS sensitive, omit apple and substitute a chopped banana after cooking)
3 cinnamon sticks
1/4 cup maple syrup

Bring hemp milk to a boil, add millet, apple, and cinnamon sticks. Simmer, covered, for 30 minutes, stirring every 10 minutes or so to prevent sticking. Add in maple syrup. Serve and enjoy!

Nutrition note: This simple and super yummy recipe tends to be gentle on the stomach and is an excellent source of iron. Millet is particularly high in magnesium, a common deficiency for those with IBD. Hemp milk is a great source of many nutrients including essential fatty acids such as omega-3 fatty acids, protein, iron, magnesium, and fiber not to mention it is also lactose-free!

Nutritional information per serving*:

Calories: 360
Total fat: 10 g
Saturated fat: 0 g
Carbohydrate: 63 g
Protein: 13.6 g

Cholesterol: 0 mg
Sodium: 20 mg
Dietary fiber: 5.4 g
Sugars: 24 g

*Nutritionals will vary depending on the brand of hemp milk you use, which can differ greatly.
Source: Cheryl Harris, MPH, RD, LD, *www.harriswholehealth.com*, originally created March 2009.

Side Dishes

 ## Butternut Squash and Parmesan Risotto

Makes 6 1½-cup servings

1 (2-lb.) butternut squash, peeled and cubed in 1" chunks
4 Tbsp. olive oil or vegetable oil
1 tsp. dried rosemary
6 cups chicken stock
1½ cups Arborio rice
½ cup dry white wine optional
4 cups fresh baby spinach
½ cup reduced-lactose, low-fat milk
¼ cup freshly grated Parmesan cheese

Preheat oven to 400 degrees.

Combine butternut squash, 2 tablespoons oil, and rosemary on a jellyroll (cookie sheet) pan and place in oven. Roast squash 20–30 minutes or until fork tender. Set aside.

Meanwhile, in large saucepan over medium heat, add chicken stock to keep warm.

While stock is heating up, combine 2 tablespoons of oil and rice in large non-stick skillet over medium heat. Stir frequently and cook for 2 minutes. Add wine to rice and simmer for another minute.

Using a ladle, start adding ½ cup of chicken stock at a time to the rice and stir. Continue to add stock to rice, and stir when the previous amount has been absorbed. When all stock has been added and absorbed, add spinach and lower heat to low. Stir in milk and cook for an additional minute. Gently fold in squash and garnish with Parmesan cheese. Enjoy!

Nutrition note: This is a delightful and hearty FODMAPs-friendly dish. It is a great source of calories, carbs, and protein as well as vitamins C and A, iron, and calcium.

Nutritional information per serving:

Calories: 353
Total fat: 11g
Saturated fat: 2 g
Carbohydrate: 53 g
Protein: 8 g
Cholesterol: 4 mg
Sodium: 233 mg
Dietary fiber: 4 g
Sugars: 5 g

Source: Kate Scarlata, RD, LDN, *www.katescarlata.com*, adopted from *The Complete Idiot's Guide to Eating Well With IBS* (Alpha 2010)

Quinoa with Red Pepper and Pine Nuts

Makes 6 ½-cup servings

1 cup quinoa, rinsed and drained
2 cups water
1 Tbsp. olive oil or vegetable oil

1 Tbsp. butter or trans fat–free margarine
1 medium red bell pepper, cut in strips
1 medium celery stalk, diced
¼ cup pine nuts, toasted

In medium saucepan combine quinoa and water and bring to boil over high heat. Reduce heat to low and cook covered for 15 minutes or until liquid is absorbed and quinoa is tender.

Meanwhile in large skillet, combine oil, butter, red pepper, and celery over medium heat. Cook while stirring for about 5 minutes, until vegetables are fork tender.

Add cooked quinoa to skillet and gently mix. Garnish with pine nuts. Enjoy immediately.

Nutrition note: This FODMAP-friendly recipe is made with quinoa, which is known as a rich protein grain and is delicious with the peppers and pine nuts. It is an excellent source of vitamin C as well as good source of vitamin A and iron.

Nutritional information per serving:

Calories: 186
Total fat: 9.6 g
Saturated fat: 1.7 g
Carbohydrate: 20 g
Protein: 5 g
Cholesterol: 5 mg
Sodium: 26 mg
Dietary fiber: 2.6 g
Sugars: 1.2 g

Source: Kate Scarlata, RD, LDN, *www.katescarlata.com*, adopted from *The Complete Idiot's Guide to Eating Well With IBS* (Alpha 2010)

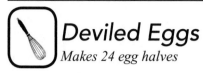

Deviled Eggs
Makes 24 egg halves

12 large eggs
4 Tbsp. mayonnaise
2 tsp. mustard

Place eggs in a 4-quart saucepan and cover them with cold water.

Bring water to a rolling boil. Turn off heat, and let eggs sit in boiled water for 20 minutes.

Drain off hot water, and rinse eggs several times in cold water.

Fill egg pan with cold water. Gently squeeze each egg until shell is crushed enough to let water seep in. Let the eggs sit in cold water for a few minutes, then remove and discard shells.

Halve each egg with a sharp knife. Collect egg yolks in a bowl, and set egg whites aside.

Mash egg yolks, mayonnaise, and mustard together until very smooth. Season with salt and pepper to taste.

Add more mayonnaise or mustard to taste.

Fill the egg white halves with spoonfuls of egg yolk mixture.

If desired, garnish the eggs with a sprinkling of paprika or little dabs of mustard.

Cover and chill until serving.

Nutrition note: This old favorite is FODMAP friendly and a great source of calories and protein. Whole-grain Dijon mustard adds a delightful flavor and some visual interest to this recipe.

Nutritional information per serving (2 egg halves):

Calories: 91
Total fat: 6.6 g
Saturated fat: 1.8 g

Carbohydrate: 1.6 g
Protein: 6.4 g
Cholesterol: 213 mg
Sodium: 114 mg
Dietary fiber: 0.03 g
Sugars: 0.71 g

Source: Patsy Catsos, MS, RD, LD, *www.ibsfree.net*, from *IBS- Free at Last! Second Edition* (Pond Cove Press, forthcoming January 2012)

Desserts

Vanilla Meringue Cookies
Makes 26 cookies

3 eggs, at room temperature
¼ tsp. cream of tartar
¾ cup superfine sugar*
¼ tsp. pure vanilla extract
½ cup mini semisweet chocolate chips (may contain some FODMAPs), optional

Preheat oven to 300 degrees.

In a small bowl, crack eggs and remove egg yolks, leaving egg whites. This can be done easily by cracking open the egg over a bowl, and allowing the whites to fall into the bowl while moving the yolk from one eggshell half to the other. Add cream of tartar to egg whites. With an electric mixer beat on medium to high speed, beat mixture until soft peaks form (mixture will be able to curl when you pull the beater up) about 2 minutes.

Slowly add sugar to egg whites ¼ cup at a time along with vanilla, and mixture will become even stiffer. Fold in chocolate chips and drop meringues by the heaping teaspoonful onto non-stick cookie sheet about 2 inches apart.

Place cookie sheet in oven then immediately reduce the heat to 200 degrees. Bake for 2 hours. Cookies will be crispy and light. Remove and cool completely. These cookies are best enjoyed within the first day of cooking.

*Can buy this type of sugar packaged. It is sugar that has been ground into smaller granular so it incorporates easier.

Nutrition Note: Light with a hint of vanilla, these airy cookies are FODMAP-friendly as well as low in calories and fat. Try adding some mini chocolate chips for a different flavor; just go easy on the chocolate.

Nutritional information per serving (2 cookies):

Calories: 80
Total fat: 1 g
Saturated fat: 1 g
Carbohydrate: 16 g
Protein: 1 g
Cholesterol: 0 mg
Sodium: 12 mg
Sugars: 16 g

Source: Kate Scarlata, RD, LDN, *www.katescarlata.com*, adopted from *The Complete Idiot's Guide to Eating Well With IBS* (Alpha 2010)

 ## Almond Shortbread Sand Dollars

Makes 24 cookies

½ cup unsalted butter
1 cup oat flour, loosely packed
1 cup almond meal flour, loosely packed
½ cup granulated sugar
1 large egg

1 tsp. vanilla extract

1 tsp. pure almond extract (no substitution)

Preheat oven to 300 degrees.

Place butter in a medium sized, microwave-safe mixing bowl; microwave 30 seconds.

Add remaining ingredients and stir together with a wooden spoon until a soft dough is formed.

Drop heaping teaspoons of dough onto un-greased cookie sheets.

Bake 20–30 minutes, until golden brown on the edges and firm to the touch.

Remove from the oven, and use a spatula to transfer the cookies to a paper towel.

Allow cookies to cool for 30 minutes, then store in an airtight container.

Nutrition note: These FODMAP-friendly cookies are delicious and even give you a boost of protein for dessert. If you are looking to gain weight, these can be quite helpful. You can use this recipe with or without the egg.

Nutritional information per serving (2 cookies):

Calories: 193

Total fat: 13 g

Saturated fat: 5.4 g

Carbohydrate: 16.7 g

Cholesterol: 38 mg

Sodium: 9 mg

Dietary fiber: 1.6 g

Sugars: 8.8 g

Source: Patsy Catsos, MS, RD, LD, *www.ibsfree.net*, from *IBS- Free at Last! Second Edition* (Pond Cove Press, Forthcoming January 2012)

Resource Guide

Books/Cookbooks/Recipes

Janssen Biotech, Inc. Living With Crohn's Disease Recipes
livingwithcrohnsdisease.com/
livingwithcrohnsdisease/life_with_crohns/recipes.html

Roberta L. Duyff, MS, RD, FADA, CFCS, and The American Dietetic Association
Authors: *American Dietetic Association Complete Food and Nutrition Guide* (Wiley 2006, next edition forthcoming 2012)

Jo Ann Hattner, MPH, RD, and Susan Anderes, MLIS
Authors: *Gut Insight* (Hattner Nutrition, 2009)

Heidi McIndoo, MS RD LDN
Author: *When to Eat What* (Adams Media, 2010)
www.appleadaynutrition.net

Victoria Shanta Retelny, RD, LDN
Author: *The Essential Guide to Healthy Healing Foods* (Alpha Books/Penguin, July 2011)
www.livingwellcommunications.com

Kate Scarlata, RD, LDN
> Author: *The Complete Idiot's Guide to Eating Well with IBS* (Alpha 2010)
> *www.katescarlata.com*

Amber J. Tresca, About.com Guide
> Recipes That Go Easy on Your IBD
> *ibdcrohns.about.com/od/dietandnutrition/a/eatibd.htm*

Elisa Zied, MS, RD, CDN
> Author: *Nutrition At Your Fingertips* (Alpha, Nov. 2009)
> Co-Author: *Feed Your Family Right!* (Wiley, 2007) and *So What Can I Eat?!* (Wiley, 2006)
> *www.elisazied.com*

Celiac Disease/Gluten-Free Diet

National Foundation For Celiac Awareness
> *www.celiaccentral.org,* accessed Feb.–March 2011

Celiac Disease Foundation
> *www.celiac.org,* accessed Feb.–March 2011

Celiac.com
> *www.celiac.com,* accessed Feb.–March 2011

Harris Whole Health/ Cheryl Harris, MPH, RD, LD
> *www.harriswholehealth.com,* accessed April 2011

Complementary and Alternative Therapies

Reiki

International Association of Reiki Professionals
> *www.iarp.org,* accessed June 2011

The International Center for Reiki Training
> *www.reiki.org,* accessed June 2011

Yoga

Yoga Basics
> *yogabasics.com,* accessed June 2011

Yoga Journal
> *www.yogajournal.com,* accessed June 2011

Acupuncture

Acupuncture.com
> *www.acupunture.com,* accessed June 2011

National Certification Commission for Acupuncture and American Academy of Medical Acupuncture
> *www.medicalacupunture.org,* accessed June 2011

Oriental Medicine
> *www.nccaom.org,* accessed June 2011

Dietitians Specializing in Digestive Disorders

Patsy Catsos, MS, RD, LD
> Portland, ME
> *www.ibsfree.net*
> E-mail: patsycatsos@gmail.com
> Author: *IBS—Free at Last!* (Second Edition)
> *The Revolutionary, New Step-by-Step Method for Those Who Have Tried Everything. Control IBS Symptoms by Limiting FODMAPS Carbohydrates in Your Diet* (forthcoming Pond Cove Press, 2012)

Cheryl Harris, MPH, RD, LD
> Harris Whole Health
> Alexandria, VA
> *www.harrishealth.com*
> Twitter: @cherylharrisrd

Angela Hermes, RD, CLT
Wellness and Nutrition Coach
www.NourishingTransitions.com

Gita Patel, MS, RD, CDE, LD, CLT
Author, Consultant, Speaker
www.feedinghealth.com
E-mail: gita@feedinghealth.com

Jan Patenaude, RD
Certified LEAP Therapist
Director of Medical Nutrition
Signet Diagnostic Corp.
www.betterbloodtest.com
E-mail: DineRight4@aol.com

Kate Scarlata, RD, LDN
Boston, Mass
www.katescarlata.com
twitter.com/beegood
Author: *The Complete Idiot's Guide to Eating Well
with IBS* (Alpha 2010)

Digestive Disorder Websites

American College of Gastroenterology
www.acg.gi.org, accessed Feb.–April 2011

American Gastroenterological Association
hwww.gastro.org, accessed Feb.–April 2011

American Society of Colon and Rectal Surgeons
www.fascrs.org, accessed Feb.–April 2011

**International Foundation for Functional
Gastrointestinal Disorders**
www.iffgd.org, accessed Feb.–April 2011

National Digestive Diseases Information Clearinghouse, NIDDK, NIH
> *digestive.niddk.nih.gov,* accessed Feb.–April 2011

Diverticular Disease

Diverticulosis
> *diverticulosis.org,* accessed April 2011

UCSF Medical Center/Diverticular Disease and Diet
> *www.ucsfhealth.org/education/diverticular_disease_and_diet/,* accessed April 2011

WebMD/ Digestive Disorders Health Center/ Diverticulosis
> *www.webmd.com/digestive-disorders/tc/diverticulosis-topic-overview,* accessed April 2011

Healthy Eating

American Dietetic Association
> *www.eatright.org,* accessed June 2011

USDA Dietary Guidelines for Americans 2010
> *www.cnpp.usda.gov/dietaryguidelines.htm,* accessed June 2011

USDA Choosemyplate.gov
> *www.choosemyplate.gov,* accessed June 2011

What You Need to Know about Mercury in Fish and Shellfish
> U.S. Environmental Protection Agency, EPA
> *water.epa.gov/scitech/swguidance/fishshellfish/outreach/advice_index.cfm,* accessed June 2011

Herbs/Dietary Supplements

Herbs at a Glance: A Quick Guide to Herbal Supplements (National Center for Complementary and Alternative Medicine)
nccam.nih.gov/health/NIH_Herbs_at_a_Glance.pdf, accessed June 2011

Herb Research Foundation
www.herbs.org, accessed June 2011

National Center for Complementary and Alternative Medicine
nccam.nih.gov/health/supplements/wiseuse.htm, accessed June 2011

National Institutes for Health/Office of Dietary Supplements
ods.od.nih.gov, accessed June 2011

Natural Medicines Comprehensive Database
naturaldatabase.therapeuticresearch.com, accessed June 2011

United States National Library of Medicine Dietary Supplements Labels Database
dietarysupplements.nlm.nih.gov/dietary/, accessed June 2011

Inflammatory Bowel Disease (IBD)

About.com Inflammatory Bowel Disease (IBD)
Amber J. Tresca, Inflammatory Bowel Disease (IBD) Guide
ibdcrohns.about.com, accessed Feb.–June 2011

Crohn's & Colitis Foundation of America
www.ccfa.org/info/about/crohns, accessed Feb.–June 2011

Crohn's Disease Free
www.crohnsdiseasefree.com, accessed Feb.–June 2011

Crohn's Online
www.crohnsdiseasefree.com, accessed Feb.–June 2011

Health Central/ MyIBDcentral.com
> *www.healthcentral.com/ibd/,* accessed Feb.–June 2011

Kate Scarlata, RD
> FODMAPs Information and Recipes
> *katescarlata.wordpress.com/fodmaps/,* accessed Feb.–
> June 2011

WebMD-Crohn's Disease Health Center
> *www.webmd.com/ibd-crohns-disease/crohns-disease/*
> *creating-a-crohns-disease-diet-plan,* accessed
> Feb.–June 2011

WebMD-Inflammatory Bowel Disease Health Center
> *www.webmd.com/ibd-crohns-disease/default.htm,* accessed
> Feb.–June 2011

WebMD-Ulcertative Colitis Health Center
> *webmd.com/ibd-crohns-disease/ulcerative-colitis-topic-*
> *overview,* accessed Feb.–June 2011

WomensHealth.gov/Inflammatory Bowel Disease
> *www.womenshealth.gov/faq/inflammatory-bowel-disease.cfm,*
> accessed Feb.–June 2011

Specific Carbohydrate Diet (SCD) Web Library
> *www.scdiet.org/,* accessed Feb.–June 2011

Irritable Bowel Syndrome
Irritable Bowel Syndrome Self Help and Support Group
> *www.ibsgroup.org/forums*

WebMD/Irritable Bowel Syndrome (IBS) Help Center
> *www.webmd.com/ibs/default.htm*

Kids and IBD
CDHNF/Children's Digestive Health and Nutrition Foundation
> *www.cdhnf.org,* accessed March–April 2011

KidsHealth/Inflammatory Bowel Disease
 kidshealth.org/parent/medical/digestive/ibd.html#, accessed
 March–April 2011

The Pediatric IBD Foundation
 www.pedsibd.org/parents.treatments-goals.html,
 accessed March–April 2011

Support Groups, Tools, and Blogs for IBD

Crohn's and Colitis Foundation of America I'll Be Determined
 www.ibdetermined.org

Crohn's Forum
 www.crohnsforum.com/

Everyday Health/Colitis Blog
 www.everydayhealth.com/blog

HealingWell.com
 www.healingwell.com/ibd

IBD Support Foundation
 www.ibdsf.com

IBD Living/ Begin To Live Again
 www.ibdsf.com

Inflammatory Bowel Disease Support Group
 www.ibdsupportorg

Living With Crohn's Disease Blog
 Scottie Roy
 livingwithcrohnsdisease.blogspot.com

A Pain In The Gut
 ibdsupport.com

Shareable IBD Diary
 www.healthcentral.com/ibd/c/diaries

Bibliography

Books/Magazine Articles

Dalessandro, Tracie, MS, RD, CDN. *What To Eat With IBD*. New York: CMG Publishing, 2006.

Magee, Elaine, M.P.H., R.D. *Tell Me What to Eat if I Have Irritable Bowel Syndrome*. N.J.: New Page Books, 2000.

Palmer, Sharon, RD. "Cracking Myths Experts Bust Digestive Health's Top Misconceptions." *Today's Dietitian*, April 2011, pp. 24–31.

Scarlata, Kate, RD, LDN. "The FODMAPs Approach." *Today's Dietitian*, August 2010, pp. 30–34.

Steinhart, Hillaray, A., MD, MSc, FRCP. *Crohn's & Colitis Understanding and Managing IBD*. Ontario, Canada: Robert Rose, Inc., 2006.

Tessmer, Kimberly, RD, LD. *Tell Me What to Eat if I Have Celiac Disease.* Franklin Lakes, N.J.: New Page Books, 2009.

Online Articles and Websites

About.com Inflammatory Bowel Disease, *ibdcrohns.about.com/,* accessed March–June 2011.

Celiac Disease Foundation, *www.celiac.org,* accessed March–April 2011.

Children's Digestive Health and Nutrition Foundation (CDHNF), *www.cdhnf.org,* accessed April 2011.

"Crohn's Disease," NIH Publication, No. 06–3410 February 2006, *digestive.niddk.nih.gov/ddiseases/pubs/crohns/index.htm,* accessed March–April 2011.

"Crohn's Disease," Mayo Clinic Staff, *www.mayoclinic.com/ health/crohns-disease/DS00104,* accessed March–April 2011.

Dietary Guidelines for Americans, *www.health.gov/Dietaryguidelines,* accessed April 2011.

"Dietary Supplement Fact Sheet: Calcium," Office of Dietary Supplement (NIH), *ods.od.nih.gov/factsheets/Calcium-QuickFacts/,* accessed May 17, 2011.

"Dietary Supplement Fact Sheets" Office of Dietary Supplement (NIH), *ods.od.nih.gov/factsheets,* accessed May 25, 2011.

"Dietary Supplement Fact Sheet: Vitamin D," Office of Dietary Supplement (NIH), *ods.od.nih.gov/factsheets/VitaminD-HealthProfessional/#h2,* accessed May 17, 2011.

"Diverticulosis and Diverticulitis," NIH Publication No. 08–1163 July 2008, *digestive.niddk.nih.gov/ddiseases/pubs/diverticu-losis/,* accessed April 6, 2011.

"Diverticulosis - Topic Overview," WebMD Medical Reference from Healthwise, *www.webmd.com/digestive-disorders/tc/ diverticulosis-topic-overview*, accessed April 6, 2011.

"Exercise May Help Soothe Irritable Bowels", Amy Norton, *www.reuters.com/article/2011/01/12/us-irritable-bowels-idUSTRE70B70R20110112*, accessed May 16, 2011.

"Finding the Right Diet for IBS," Kathleen M. Zelman, MPH, RD, LD/WebMD Feature, *www.webmd.com/ibs/features/finding-right-diet-ibs*, accessed April, 5 2011.

"Fish and Omega-3 Fatty Acids", American Heart Association, *www.americanheart.org/presenter.jhtml?identifier=4632*, accessed June 1, 2011.

"FODMAPs," Kate Scarlata, RD, *katescarlata.wordpress.com/ fodmaps/*, accessed April 28, 2011.

Herbs Research Foundation, *www.herbs.org/herbnews/*, accessed June 2010.

"How to Stay Fit When You Have Inflammatory Bowel Disease," Alan V. Safdi, MD, FACG, *www.salix.com/patient-resources/ digestive-health-newsletter/archive/exercise-with-ibd. aspx#difference*, accessed May 16, 2011.

"Inflammatory Bowel Disease," The National Women's Health Information Center, Reviewed by: Jacqueline Wolf, M.D., *www.womenshealth.gov/faq/inflammatory-bowel-disease. cfm*, accessed March–April 2011.

Inflammatory Bowel Disease Health Center, WebMD, *www.webmd.com/ibd-crohns-disease/default.htm*, accessed March–May 2011.

"Lactose Intolerance," NIH Publication No. 09–2751, June 2009, *digestive.niddk.nih.gov/ddiseases/pubs/ lactoseintolerance/#products*, accessed May 6, 2011.

NIH Office of Dietary Supplements, *ods.od.nih.gov/*, accessed June 2011.

"Nutritional Considerations in Inflammatory Bowel Disease," Kelly Anne Eiden, M.S., R.D., CNSD, *Practical Gastroenterology,* May 2003, *www.medicine.virginia.edu/ clinical/departments/medicine/divisions/digestive-health/ nutrition-support-team/nutrition-articles/may03eidenarticle. pdf*, accessed April 2011.

SCD Web Library, *www.scdiet.org*, accessed April 28, 2011.

"The Specific Carbohydrate Diet: Does It Work?", Debra Gordon, Crohn's and Colitis Foundation of America, *www.ccfa.org/ about/news/scd*, accessed April 29, 2011.

"Ulcerative Colitis," Mayo Clinic Staff, *www.mayoclinic.com/ health/ulcerative-colitis/DS00598*, accessed March–April 2011.

"Ulcerative Colitis," NIH Publication No. 06–1597 February 2006, *digestive.niddk.nih.gov/ddiseases/pubs/colitis/index.htm*, accessed March–April 2011.

"Understanding the Goals of Treatment," Pediatric IBD Foundation, *www.pedsibd.org/parents/treatments-goals.html*, accessed April 2011.

U.S. Department of Agriculture, Agricultural Research Service, 2009. USDA National Nutrient Database for Standard Reference, Release 22. Nutrient Data Laboratory Home Page, *www.ars.usda.gov/ba/bhnrc/ndl*, accessed May 6, 2011.

USDA DRI Tables, f*nic.nal.usda.gov/nal_display/index. php?info_center=4&tax_level=3&tax_subject=256&topic_ id=1342&level3_id=5140*, accessed May 26, 2011.

USDA MyPlate.gov, *www.choosemyplate.gov*, accessed June 2, 2011.

WebMD- Crohn's Disease Health Center, *www.webmd.com/ibd-crohns-disease/Crohns-disease/creating-a-crohns-disease-diet-plan*, accessed March–June 2011.

WebMD- Ulcertative Colitis Health Center, *www.webmd.com/ibd-crohns-disease/ulcerative-colitis/ulcerative-colitis-topic-overview*, accessed March–June 2011.

WebMD- Inflammatory Bowel Disease Health Center, *www.webmd.com/ibd-crohns-disease/default.htm*, accessed March–June 2011.

"What to Eat During Flare-ups of Ulcerative Colitis," Cicely A. Richard, eHow Contributor, *www.ehow.com/ way_5251846_eat-during-flare_ups-ulcerative-colitis.html*, accessed May 1, 2011.

"What I Need to Know About Irritable Bowel Syndrome," NIH Publication No. 07–4686, May 2007, *digestive.niddk.nih.gov/ddiseases/pubs/ibs_ez/*, accessed April 5, 2011.

"What is Reiki?", The International Center for Reiki Training, *www.reiki.org/faq/whatisreiki.html*, accessed June 2011.

"What You Need to Know About Mercury in Fish and Shellfish," U.S. Environmental Protection Agency, *water.epa.gov/scitech/swguidance/fishshellfish/outreach/advice_index.cfm*, accessed June 1, 2011.

"Your Digestive System and How It Works," NIH Publication No. 08–2681, April 2008, *digestive.niddk.nih.gov/ddiseases/pubs/yrdd/*, accessed March 2011.

Index

About the Author

Kimberly A. Tessmer, RD LD, is an author and consulting dietitian in Brunswick, Ohio. Her books include: *The Complete Idiot's Guide to The Mediterranean Diet, Tell Me What to Eat If I Am Trying To Conceive, Tell Me What to Eat If I Have Celiac Disease, The Everything Nutrition Book*, and *The Everything Pregnancy Nutrition Book*. Kim currently owns and operates ***Nutrition Focus*** (*www.Nutrifocus.net*), a consulting company specializing in weight management, authoring, menu development, and other nutritional services. In addition, Kim acts as the RD on the board of directors for Lifestyles Technologies, Inc., a company that provides nutrition software solutions, developing a wide array of nutritionally sound meal templates.